COMPLETE GUIDE
OF
RED LIGHT THERAPY

Susan McDowell

COMPLETE GUIDE TO RED LIGHT THERAPY

Optimal health, healthy skin, and other benefits of red light

- Susan McDowell -

Complete guide to red light therapy / Susan McDowell – 1st Edition

ISBN 9798321451335

INDEX

CAUTION

It is important to follow general guidelines and protocols to ensure safe and effective application of red light therapy. Some practical tips include:

Consult a healthcare professional: Before beginning any red light therapy treatment, it is advisable to consult a healthcare professional, such as a physician or therapist, especially if you have any pre-existing medical conditions.

Follow the manufacturer's instructions: Each red light therapy device has its own instructions for use. It is important to read and follow these instructions carefully to ensure proper and safe use.

Establish a routine and be consistent: Red light therapy may require regular sessions for optimal results. Establishing a routine and being consistent in the application of the therapy is important to maximize its benefits.

Maintain an adequate distance: It is important to maintain an adequate distance between the red light device and the skin to ensure optimal exposure and avoid damage. By following the manufacturer's recommendations, the optimal distance can be determined for each device.

Protect the eyes: Red light can be intense and potentially harmful to the eyes. It is important to wear appropriate eye protection goggles when necessary and to avoid looking directly at the light source during therapy.

Be patient and realistic: Red light therapy can provide benefits, but results may vary depending on the individual and the condition being treated. It is important to be patient and realistic, and to maintain reasonable expectations for results.

By following these guidelines and practical tips, those who wish to explore red light therapy for themselves can do so safely and effectively, maximizing the benefits this therapy can offer. However, it is important to remember that each individual is unique, and it is advisable to seek the advice of a healthcare professional before beginning any new treatment.

It is important to note that red light therapy does not seek to replace conventional medical treatments, but rather to complement them. It is considered a non-invasive and generally safe therapy, although it is advisable to follow specific guidelines and recommendations for proper use.

Medical consultation and thorough research is strongly recommended for treatment and impact it may have on each condition and on an individual basis.

INTRODUCTION TO RED LIGHT THERAPY

The application of red and near-infrared light produces a chain reaction, stimulating collagen production and improving blood circulation. Superficially, this can accelerate the healing of wounds, such as burns or ulcers, and reduce signs of aging, such as wrinkles and dark spots.

Although the skin is the largest and most visible organ of the body, theoretically all cells can benefit from red or near-infrared light therapy.

In general, the tissues that benefit the most are those in a state of depletion or alteration, such as skin damaged by the sun. Although phototherapy is not a miracle solution for treating skin or any other condition, it does offer numerous advantages that make this practice considered, if not an ideal complement to other treatments, a form of prevention and care in itself.

"It looks great - and I've seen it all over social media - but does red light therapy really work?" you may be asking yourself if you decided to read this book. And the answer is yes. But before we get into the details about a red light that claims to cure everything (and in a way it can), let us talk about the purpose of the book and then get into materia of what red light therapy is and why it works for skin all over the body, among other benefits.

THE OBJECTIVE OF THE BOOK

The purpose of this book is to provide an accessible and understandable guide to red light therapy, an innovative therapeutic approach that has gained recognition and popularity in recent years. Our goal is to provide clear and concise information on the fundamentals of red light therapy, its potential benefits and its various applications in the health and wellness field.

In a world where health and wellbeing are constantly evolving, it is essential that information about therapeutic approaches such as red light therapy be accessible to all. This book aims to fill that gap, presenting the subject in a clear and understandable way to a wide audience.

Red light therapy has shown significant benefits in a variety of conditions and conditions, but there is still some confusion and lack of information about its operation and application. That is why it is crucial to address this topic in an informative format, so that both health professionals and the general public can understand the basic concepts and explore the possibilities that this therapy offers.

This book seeks to be a reliable and comprehensive source of information about red light therapy, providing an overview of its scientific foundations, its history, its contemporary applications, and its future potential. In addition, we will present research and testimonials that support its efficacy and clinical relevance, providing a solid basis for understanding and considering red light therapy as a viable therapeutic option.

By addressing red light therapy in an informative format, we hope this book will inspire readers to explore this therapeutic approach, either as health professionals seeking new therapeutic tools or as individuals interested in improving their health and wellbeing. We are convinced that clear and accessible information can empower people to make informed decisions about their well-being, and we are committed to providing them with the tools they need to do so.

Red light therapy is a therapeutic approach that uses light in the red spectrum to promote health and well-being. This form of therapy is based on the idea that exposure to low-intensity red light can have beneficial effects on biological tissues and trigger positive responses in the body.

Red light used in red light therapy has a specific wavelength, usually in the range of 600 to 700 nanometers. This particular wavelength is able to penetrate the deeper layers of the skin and reach the underlying tissues, where it can interact with cells and biological systems.

One of the main benefits of red light therapy is its ability to stimulate energy production in cells through mitochondrial activation, known as photobiomodulation. This process triggers a series of biochemical and bioelectric responses that can have positive effects on different systems of the body.

Common benefits associated with red light therapy include:

Improving wound healing and tissue regeneration: Red light has been shown to speed up the wound healing process, stimulate collagen production and improve the regeneration of damaged tissue.

Pain relief and reduction of inflammation: Red light therapy can have analgesic and anti-inflammatory effects, helping to reduce pain and inflammation in various conditions, such as muscle injuries, arthritis, and chronic pain.

Stimulation of blood circulation: Red light can improve blood circulation by dilating blood vessels and increasing blood flow to tissues, which favors the delivery of oxygen and nutrients needed for optimal cellular health.

Improving skin health: Red light therapy is widely used in skin care, as it can stimulate collagen production, improve skin texture, reduce wrinkles and expression lines, and treat conditions such as acne and rosacea.

Strengthening the immune system: Exposure to red light can improve the immune response by stimulating production of immune cells and promoting increased phagocytic activity, which helps fight infections and strengthen the immune system.

Red light therapy has gained relevance in the therapeutic and wellness field due to its potential to improve the health and functioning of the body in a non-invasive manner and free of significant side effects. Its application ranges from medicine and physiotherapy to dermatology and personal care.

The ability of red light to interact with cells and biological systems has sparked great interest in the scientific community, and numerous studies have supported its effectiveness in different medical and aesthetic conditions. As research continues, red light therapy is expected to continue to evolve and expand into new areas of application and discovery.

In short, red light therapy is a promising therapeutic approach that uses low-intensity red light to promote health and well-being. Benefits include improved wound healing, pain relief, stimulation of blood circulation, improved skin health, and strengthening of the immune system. Its relevance in the therapeutic and wellness field lies in its ability to offer a safe and effective alternative to other therapeutic approaches, providing notable benefits without significant side effects.

Educating and raising awareness about red light therapy is a crucial aspect to promote an accurate and objective understanding of this form of therapy. In this section, a detailed explanation of the scientific foundations and mechanisms of action of red light therapy will be provided, as well as a demystification of common misconceptions or misunderstandings related to this therapy.

Red light therapy is based on sound scientific principles and has been the subject of numerous studies and research. Its effectiveness is mainly attributed to a process known as photobiomodulation, in which low-intensity red light interacts with biological cells and tissues, triggering beneficial biochemical and bioelectric responses.

The red light used in this therapy has a specific wavelength in the range of 600 to 700 nanometers, which has been shown to be optimal for penetrating the skin and reaching the deeper layers where the target cells and tissues are located. When cells are exposed to red light, specific receptors are activated in the mitochondria, the structures responsible for the production of cellular energy.

One of the main mechanisms of action of red light therapy is the stimulation of the production of adenosine triphosphate (ATP), the main source of energy in cells. Red light increases the activity of the electron transport chain in mitochondria, leading to increased generation of ATP. This additional energy promotes cellular function and promotes a number of beneficial responses in the body.

In addition to ATP production, red light therapy also triggers other beneficial effects. For example, red light has been shown to reduce free radical production and oxidative stress in cells, contributing to reduced inflammation and cell damage. It has also been shown to stimulate the release of growth factors, such as insulin-like growth factor (IGF-1), which promotes tissue regeneration and repair.

It is important to address some common misconceptions or misunderstandings related to red light therapy. One is the idea that red light therapy is similar to excessive exposure to ultraviolet (UV) radiation from the sun or tanning beds. It is noteworthy that red light therapy uses a specific wavelength that does not cause thermal damage or skin burns. In addition, a low, controlled intensity is used to prevent adverse effects.

Another common misunderstanding is the belief that red-light therapy is just a "placebo" or pseudo-scientific approach without solid scientific backing. However, there is a substantial scientific basis supporting the benefits of red light therapy, with numerous studies and reviews

The methods and devices used to administer red light therapy shall be described, as well as general guidelines and protocols for their safe and effective application. In addition, practical advice will be offered for those who wish to begin their experience with red light therapy themselves.

Different methods and devices are available to administer red light therapy, and the choice will depend on the area of application and individual preferences.

It will also summarize relevant scientific research supporting the benefits of red light therapy, as well as real testimonials from people who have experienced significant benefits through its use.

WHAT IS RED LIGHT THERAPY

Red light therapy is a therapeutic modality that uses light in the red spectrum range to promote health and wellbeing benefits. This form of therapy is based on the idea that exposure to red light can stimulate biological processes in the body, which in turn can have positive effects in various physiological conditions and functions.

The main goal of red light therapy is to harness the specific properties of light in the red range to trigger beneficial biological responses in the human body. Through controlled exposure to red light, we seek to stimulate different systems and tissues to promote healing, improve physical and mental performance, and optimize overall health.

The red light used in this therapy usually has a wavelength between about 600 and 700 nanometers, which corresponds to the visible portion of the electromagnetic spectrum. At this wavelength, red light can penetrate deep into biological tissues, reaching the underlying cells and organs.

Red light therapy has been used in various applications, including mood disorders such as depression and anxiety, sleep disorders, dermatological conditions, muscle and joint injuries, and wound healing processes, among others.

Red light used in red light therapy is a form of electromagnetic radiation that is at the visible end of the light spectrum. It has a longer wavelength compared to blue or ultraviolet light, which gives it particular properties and specific effects on biological tissues.

Properties of red light:

Wavelength: Red light has a wavelength of approximately 600 to 700 nanometers, making it longer than other parts of the visible spectrum.

Penetration: Red light can penetrate deeper into biological tissues compared to blue or ultraviolet light. It can reach underlying cells, tissues, and organs, making it suitable for therapeutic applications.

Energy: Red light has a lower energy than ultraviolet light, which makes it less harmful to skin and tissues.

Interaction of red light with biological tissues:

Absorption: When red light reaches biological tissues, some of it is absorbed by molecules present in cells, such as cytochrome c oxidase and mitochondrial chromophores. These molecules have a high affinity for red light and can absorb it, triggering specific biological responses.

Metabolic stimulation: Absorption of red light by molecules in cells can increase production of adenosine triphosphate (ATP), the cellular energy source. This can stimulate cell metabolism and promote enzyme activity.

Improved blood circulation: Red light can stimulate the release of nitric oxide into blood vessels, which causes vasodilation and improves local blood circulation. This can facilitate the delivery of oxygen and nutrients to tissues and promote the disposal of waste products.

Mechanisms of action involved in red light therapy include modulation of gene expression, reduction of inflammation, promotion of collagen and elastin synthesis, regulation of the circadian cycle, and improvement of mitochondrial function.

Red light used in red light therapy has specific properties, such as its wavelength and penetration capacity, that distinguish it from other parts of the electromagnetic spectrum. When it interacts with biological tissues, red light is absorbed by molecules and triggers a number of beneficial biological responses, such as metabolic stimulation and improved blood circulation. These mechanisms of action are fundamental to understanding the therapeutic effects of red light therapy.

In addition to the mechanisms mentioned above, there are other important biological processes that are involved in the interaction of red light with biological tissues during red light therapy:

Production of reactive oxygen species (ROS):

Exposure to red light may increase the production of ROS in cells. These molecules, such as hydrogen peroxide, can trigger cellular responses, such as activation of signaling pathways and modulation of gene expression.

Controlled generation of ROS can have beneficial effects, such as stimulating endogenous antioxidant response and promoting cell repair.

Modulation of cellular signaling pathways:

Red light can influence a variety of cell signaling pathways including the insulin-like growth factor (IGF-1) pathway, nerve growth factor (NGF) pathway, and vascular endothelial growth factor (VEGF) pathway. These pathways are involved in the regulation of key processes, such as cell proliferation, cell survival, and angiogenesis.

Modulation of these signaling pathways can have positive effects on tissue regeneration, reduction of inflammation, and promotion of healing.

Importantly, the exact mechanisms of action of red light therapy are still being investigated and understood in detail. There are several theories and approaches in the scientific literature, and the interaction of red light with biological tissues is an active field of research.

Understanding these physical fundamentals and mechanisms of action is essential to properly apply red light therapy under different conditions and optimize its therapeutic effects. As research in this field progresses, a more complete understanding of the biological processes involved and their clinical implications is expected, which may lead to a better use of red light therapy in therapeutic practice.

Red light therapy has its roots in scientific research into the effects of light on living organisms. Over the years, studies and experiments have been conducted that have contributed to its discovery and development

In the 19th century, the Danish physicist Niels Ryberg Finsen carried out pioneering research on the effects of light on the treatment of diseases. Finsen was awarded the Nobel Prize in Medicine in 1903 for his studies on the use of light therapy in the treatment of cutaneous tuberculosis, using special lamps that emitted red light.

During the 20th century, further research was conducted on the effects of red light on biological processes. It was found that red light could have beneficial effects on wound healing, stimulating hair growth, improving cognitive function and mood regulation.

The therapeutic use of red light received a significant boost with the development of laser technologies in the 1960s. Low-power lasers and LED light sources began to be used in red light therapy, allowing for more precise and controlled application.

In the 1990s, there was a significant growth in the research and application of red light therapy. Clinical studies and experiments were conducted in various application areas, such as mood disorders, sleep disorders, wound healing, and dermatological conditions.

From the 2000s onwards, red light therapy has continued to evolve and expand in various areas. Portable and home-use devices have been developed that allow people to perform red light therapy in the comfort of their homes. In addition, research has been carried out on the optimization of treatment protocols, the combination of red light with other therapeutic approaches and the exploration of new potential applications.

The evolution of red light therapy has been driven by technological advances and scientific research in several fields. As the understanding of the mechanisms of action and biological effects of red light has deepened, new applications have been discovered and treatment protocols refined. Some important developments in red light therapy include advances in light source technology. The availability of low-power lasers and high-quality light-emitting diodes (LEDs) has enabled precise and controlled red light emission in therapeutic applications. In addition, the miniaturization and portability of red-light devices have made them easier to use at home and in clinical settings.

Clinical studies and scientific evidence have also been developed. Red light therapy has been backed by a growing body of scientific evidence. Controlled clinical studies and clinical trials have been conducted to evaluate its efficacy in various medical conditions. This has contributed to its recognition and acceptance in the field of medicine and physical therapy. And obviously in combination with other therapies. Red light therapy has been combined with other therapies, such as conventional physical therapy, photodynamic therapy, and drug therapy. These combinations may improve treatment outcomes by exploiting the synergistic effects of different treatment modalities.

In cosmetic and beauty applications, red light therapy has gained popularity in the field of aesthetics and skin care. It has been used to improve the appearance of the skin, reduce wrinkles, and fine lines, and stimulate the production of collagen and elastin. It has also been used in hair treatments to promote hair growth and improve scalp health.

It is currently in the process of research into new areas of application. In addition to established applications, red light therapy is being explored in new areas. This includes potential use in neurodegenerative disorders, eye diseases, sleep disorders, musculoskeletal conditions, and metabolic disorders. Research continues to expand the limits of its application and discover new therapeutic benefits.

Red light therapy has evolved from its earliest discoveries into a recognized and widely used therapy in various fields. Technological advances, scientific research and the accumulation of clinical evidence have driven its development and application in a wide range of medical and aesthetic conditions. As new findings are discovered and new application areas are explored, red light therapy will continue to evolve and contribute to the field of medicine and physical therapy.

Red light therapy has been associated with a wide variety of therapeutic benefits in various application areas. Listed below are some of the potential therapeutic benefits of red light therapy:

1-   Improved mood and mood disorders:

Exposure to red light has been shown to be effective in treating mood disorders, such as seasonal depression and other types of depression.

Red light therapy can help regulate circadian rhythms, stimulate production of serotonin (a neurotransmitter associated with well-being), and reduce symptoms of depression and anxiety.

2-   Sleep disorders and circadian rhythm regulation:

Red light can help regulate the circadian rhythm, promoting better sleep quality and relief of sleep disorders, such as insomnia.

Exposure to red light at specific times of day can help synchronize the body's internal clock and promote healthy sleep.

3-   Improving tissue healing and regeneration:

Red light therapy has been shown to accelerate wound healing, promoting cell proliferation, new blood vessel formation, and collagen synthesis.

It has been used in the treatment of burns, ulcers, post-surgical wounds, and sports injuries to promote faster healing and reduce inflammation.

4-   Skin Care and Rejuvenation:

Red light stimulates the production of collagen and elastin in the skin, improving the appearance of wrinkles, fine lines, and sagging.

It has been used in the treatment of acne, rosacea, and other dermatological conditions to reduce inflammation, promote healing, and improve the overall appearance of the skin.

5-   Pain relief and reduction of inflammation:

Red light therapy can have analgesic and anti-inflammatory effects, relieving pain and reducing inflammation in various conditions, such as arthritis, muscle, and joint injuries.

It has been used in physical therapy and rehabilitation to speed recovery and reduce pain associated with injuries and chronic conditions.

6-   Improving sports performance and recovery:

Red light therapy can help improve muscle recovery, reduce recovery time after strenuous exercise, and promote muscle regeneration.

It has been used in athletes and athletes to improve performance, reduce fatigue, and accelerate muscle recovery.

These are just a few examples of the potential therapeutic benefits associated with red light therapy. It is important to note that individual effectiveness and response may vary depending on the medical condition and the person. It is always advisable to consult with a health professional before initiating any red light therapy treatment.

In addition to the therapeutic benefits mentioned above, red light therapy has also shown potential in other application areas. Here are some additional examples:

Treatment of neurodegenerative disorders: The effects of red light therapy on neurodegenerative diseases such as Alzheimer's and Parkinson's are being investigated. It has been suggested that red light may have neuroprotective properties and promote neuronal regeneration.

Improving eye health: Red light therapy is being explored as a treatment option for eye conditions such as age-related macular degeneration and glaucoma. Red light is thought to have positive effects on blood circulation and cell regeneration in ocular tissues.

Improved cognitive function: Red light therapy has been shown to improve cognitive function, including memory, focus, and concentration. This can be beneficial in academic, work and sports performance.

Support in metabolic disorders: Use of red light therapy in the treatment of metabolic disorders, such as obesity and insulin resistance, is being investigated. Red light is thought to influence cellular metabolism and hormonal regulation.

It is remarkable that red light therapy is not a miracle cure for all diseases and conditions. While it has shown promising benefits in several areas, more scientific research is needed to fully understand its mechanisms of action and its effectiveness under different conditions.

Red light therapy can be administered by a variety of methods and devices, each of which has its own specific characteristics and applications. The following are common methods used to administer red light therapy:

1-   Personal use red light devices: These devices are portable and designed for personal use at home or in clinical settings. They may include red-light lamps, light panels, hand-held therapy devices, or topical devices, such as red-light face masks. These devices typically emit low to medium intensity red light and can be used on specific areas of the body or face.

2-   Red Light Therapy Booths: Booths are enclosed structures equipped with multiple red light sources. The patient is placed inside the cabin to receive widespread exposure of red light throughout the body. This approach is useful when more extensive exposure is required and is used in clinical settings or red light therapy spas.

3-   Low power lasers: Low power lasers emit red light in the form of a focused beam. These lasers can be used by health care practitioners in more specific treatments, such as targeted therapy in areas of pain, wounds, or specific tissues. Low-powered lasers are commonly used in physical therapy and rehabilitation.

While red light therapy protocols may vary depending on the medical condition and device used, there are some general guidelines that can be followed:

Session duration: Red light therapy sessions usually last between 10 and 30 minutes, depending on the condition and the device used. It is important to follow the device manufacturer's recommendations or the health care practitioner's instructions.

Treatment frequency: Red light therapy is often given several times per week, with an initial treatment regimen followed by long-term maintenance. Frequency may vary depending on the condition and individual response to treatment.

Distance and exposure time: The distance between the red light device and the treatment area may vary depending on the device and desired intensity. In general, it is recommended to place the device at a distance that allows for comfortable and safe exposure. The exposure time may also vary, but it is important to avoid overexposure to red light.

Use of eye protection: In some cases, especially when using low-powered lasers, the use of eye protection is recommended to avoid direct exposure to light. This may include wearing specific protective glasses.

It is essential to follow the device manufacturer's instructions and, in case of doubt, consult with a healthcare professional trained in red light therapy. Each condition and situation may require a specific approach and protocol, so it is important to receive professional guidance.

It is important that red light therapy is generally safe and non-invasive. However, some precautions and contraindications may apply in certain cases. General considerations include medical consultation, dose review, and selective photobiomodulation.

It is always advisable to consult a doctor or health professional before starting red light therapy, especially if you have any pre-existing medical condition or are under medical treatment. It is essential to follow the specific dose and exposure time recommendations provided by the device manufacturer or healthcare professional. The recommended exposure time should not be exceeded, as overexposure can have adverse effects. Some conditions may require specific red light therapy protocols that include different wavelengths, intensities, and exposure times. It is important to adjust the parameters according to the specific treatment needs.

Caution is important under certain conditions. Red light therapy may not be suitable for people with acute eye disorders, skin cancer, extreme sensitivity to light, or thyroid disorders. In such cases, it is important to seek the opinion of a doctor before starting treatment.

Remember that red light therapy is a complementary form of treatment and does not replace conventional medical advice or treatment. It is important to use it as part of a comprehensive approach to health care and under the supervision of trained professionals.

Red light therapy has gained recognition and relevance in the therapeutic field due to its potential to complement and improve other forms of treatment. The importance of red light therapy in the therapeutic context is discussed below:

Supplementing other treatments: Red light therapy has been used in complementary ways in combination with other therapeutic approaches, such as physical therapy, psychotherapy, and medication. In many cases, red light therapy has been shown to enhance outcomes and accelerate healing processes. As it is non-invasive and safe, it can be used in conjunction with other treatments without interfering with them.

Synergistic effects: Red light therapy has been shown to have synergistic effects with other therapeutic approaches. For example, it has been used with physical therapy to relieve pain and promote recovery from muscle and joint injuries. It has also been combined with cognitive-behavioral therapy in the treatment of mood disorders to improve depressive and anxiety symptoms.

Wide range of applications: Red light therapy has proven effective in a wide range of medical conditions and disorders, making it relevant in various therapeutic specialties. From sleep disorders and mood disorders to skin problems and wound healing, red light therapy has been used in a variety of clinical settings and has shown positive results.

Research and testimonials support its efficacy and clinical relevance. There is a growing body of scientific research supporting the efficacy and clinical relevance of red light therapy in various conditions. Controlled clinical studies have shown efficacy in relieving pain, improving blood circulation, stimulating cell regeneration, and reducing inflammation. This research supports the application of red light therapy in different therapeutic fields.

In turn, many patients have shared positive testimonials about the benefits they have experienced with red light therapy. They have reported a reduction in pain, improvement in mood, faster wound healing, and improvement in sleep quality, among other results. These testimonials support the clinical relevance of red light therapy and its positive impact on people's lives.

It is important to note that while red light therapy has shown benefits in several studies and testimonials, more research is needed to fully understand its mechanisms of action and its effectiveness under different conditions. Healthcare professionals are encouraged to continue to research and use red light therapy responsibly and based on available scientific evidence.

Red light therapy plays a key role in the therapeutic context by supplementing other forms of treatment and providing additional benefits. Its ability to improve blood circulation, stimulate cell regeneration and reduce inflammation makes it a relevant therapeutic option in a wide range of medical conditions. Scientific research and patient testimonies support its efficacy and clinical relevance. However, it is critical that health care practitioners continue to responsibly investigate and apply red light therapy, following established guidelines and recommendations.

HISTORY OF RED LIGHT THERAPY

Understanding the effects of light on biological tissues has been a process that has evolved throughout history. From early indications that light could have an impact on living organisms to pioneering experiments that explored its effects on tissue healing and regeneration, considerable progress has been made in our understanding of red light therapy.

The first indications of the effect of light on living organisms date back to ancient times. Civilizations such as ancient China and Egypt were already using sunlight for therapeutic purposes. Exposure to sunlight was thought to have healing properties and could help in the treatment of various diseases.

However, it was in the 19th century that pioneering experiments were carried out that laid the groundwork for modern understanding of the effects of light on biological tissues. One of the outstanding researchers in this field was the Danish scientist Niels Ryberg Finsen, who received the Nobel Prize in Medicine in 1903 for his contributions to light therapy in the treatment of cutaneous tuberculosis.

Finsen used carbon arc lamps and ultraviolet light to treat patients with cutaneous tuberculosis. He observed significant improvements in the patients' skin condition, leading him to conclude that light could have a therapeutic effect on biological tissues. His research laid the groundwork for future studies on the use of light in the medical context.

In addition to Finsen, other scientists also conducted experiments that explored the effects of light on tissue healing and regeneration. For example, in the 1960s, Hungarian scientist Endre Mester conducted experiments with low-powered lasers and discovered that red light could stimulate hair growth and wound healing in mice. Their findings opened new doors in research into red light therapy and its application in medicine.

These pioneering experiments laid the groundwork for the current understanding of the effects of light on biological tissues and the subsequent evolution of red light therapy. From these first indications, numerous scientific studies have been carried out and progress has been made in understanding the mechanisms of light action in biological processes, leading to the development of more sophisticated technologies and devices for the administration of red light therapy.

The discovery of the effects of light on biological tissues did not stop at pioneering experiments. Over the years, additional research has broadened our understanding of the mechanisms of action of red light therapy and explored its therapeutic applications in various areas.

In recent decades, red light has been shown to penetrate deep into biological tissues and stimulate a number of beneficial biochemical and cellular responses. Red light has been found to activate mitochondria, the structures responsible for energy production in cells, leading to stimulation of cell metabolism and release of key molecules for tissue repair and regeneration.

In addition to its effects on cell energy production, red light has also been shown to have anti-inflammatory and analgesic properties. It has been shown to reduce the production of pro-inflammatory molecules and decrease the sensitivity of pain receptors, resulting in reduced pain and inflammation under different conditions.

Red light therapy has found applications in various areas of medicine and therapy. For example, in the field of dermatology, it has been used for the treatment of skin conditions such as acne, chronic wounds and scars. It has also been used in physical therapy to speed recovery from muscle and joint injuries as well as to relieve associated pain and inflammation.

In addition, the use of red light therapy in mood disorders such as depression and seasonal affective disorder has been investigated. It has been observed that exposure to red light can have positive effects on mood, improve depressive symptoms and regulate circadian rhythms.

Remarkably, while red light therapy has demonstrated benefits in various areas, its specific application may vary depending on the individual patient's condition and needs. Careful evaluation and professional supervision are required to determine the appropriate protocol and to ensure its safety and efficacy.

The first attempts to use red light for therapeutic purposes date back to the late 19th and early 20th centuries. During this period, scientists began to explore the potential benefits of red light in the medical context and to develop techniques for its therapeutic application.

One of the first studies to explore the benefits of red light in the medical environment was conducted by Danish doctor Niels Ryberg Finsen. In the late 19th century, Finsen investigated the effects of light in the treatment of skin diseases, specifically cutaneous tuberculosis. Using carbon arc lamps and ultraviolet light, Finsen managed to improve the condition of the patients, observing a decrease in symptoms and an improvement in the healing of skin lesions.

Finsen's work was groundbreaking, and in recognition of his contributions, he was awarded the Nobel Prize in Medicine in 1903. His studies laid the groundwork for further research into red light therapy and paved the way for its application in various diseases and conditions.

Based on Finsen's studies, other researchers continued to explore the benefits of red light in the medical context. In the mid-20th century, Hungarian scientist Endre Mester conducted experiments with low-powered lasers, discovering that red light could stimulate hair growth and wound healing in mice. These findings laid the groundwork for future research on red light therapy in the field of dermatology and regenerative medicine.

In the following decades, additional studies were conducted that explored the benefits of red light in various conditions and diseases. Its effects in the treatment of pain, inflammation, muscle and joint injuries, and other dermatological conditions were investigated. These initial studies laid the groundwork for the development of more advanced treatment protocols and technologies in the field of red light therapy.

As research has progressed, our understanding of the mechanisms of action of red light and its effect on biological tissues has broadened. Technological advances have allowed the creation of more sophisticated and high-quality devices that allow for the precise and effective application of red light therapy.

The first attempts to use red light for therapeutic purposes date back to the 19th century, with the pioneering studies of Niels Ryberg Finsen. These studies laid the groundwork for further research and exploration of the benefits of red light in the medical context. Over time, progress has been made in understanding the effects of red light on biological tissues, leading to the development of more sophisticated techniques and technologies for their therapeutic application. As red light therapy has gained recognition and acceptance, additional studies have been conducted to support its efficacy and have expanded its application in various areas of medicine and therapy.

Currently, there are numerous clinical and experimental studies that support the therapeutic benefits of red light. For example, red light therapy has been shown to have positive effects on wound healing by stimulating cell proliferation and granulation tissue formation. In addition, it has been shown to improve blood circulation in tissues, which contributes to cell regeneration and repair.

In the field of dermatology, red light therapy has been used to treat conditions such as acne, wrinkles, and skin spots. Red light has antibacterial and anti-inflammatory properties, which can help reduce inflammation and redness associated with acne, as well as stimulate collagen production to improve the appearance of the skin.

The use of red light therapy in the treatment of mood disorders, such as depression and seasonal affective disorder, has been investigated. Exposure to red light can stimulate production of serotonin, a neurotransmitter involved in mood regulation, which can help relieve depressive symptoms and improve emotional well-being.

It is important to mention that while red light therapy has demonstrated benefits in various areas, each case and condition should be evaluated individually and under professional supervision. Treatment protocols may vary depending on the patient's specific clinical situation and needs. Red light therapy can be used as a complementary approach along with other forms of treatment, and careful evaluation is required to determine the most appropriate strategy.

Red light therapy has experienced significant advances over the years, driven by scientific research and technological advances. Here are some key milestones in the development of this therapy and the contributions of leading scientists and practitioners:

Early research: As mentioned earlier, the pioneering work of Danish physician Niels Ryberg Finsen in the 19th century laid the foundation for red light therapy. His studies on the effects of light on the healing of skin diseases were fundamental to further research in this area.

Laser Discovery: In 1960, Theodore Maiman developed the first laser, which allowed for consistent and controlled light emission. This breakthrough technology paved the way for the precise application of red light therapy, as lasers provided a focused, high-intensity light source.

Photobiomodulation: In the 1980s, scientist Endre Mester coined the term "photobiomodulation" to describe the biological effects of light on tissues. His research on the effects of low-power lasers on wound healing and hair growth laid the groundwork for the field of red light therapy.

Advances in devices and technologies: Over the last few decades, significant advances have been made in the design and technology of red light therapy devices. LED light sources (light emitting diode) have been developed that emit red light efficiently and accurately. These devices are safer, more compact, and more affordable, making them easier to use in both clinical and home environments.

Clinical research and scientific validation: Over time, a growing body of scientific evidence has accumulated supporting the efficacy and therapeutic benefits of red light therapy under various conditions. Controlled clinical studies have shown its effectiveness in wound healing, pain relief, improvement of muscle function, tissue regeneration and other therapeutic applications.

Contributions from leading professionals: Several scientists, doctors and health professionals have made significant contributions to the advancement of red light therapy. Among them are Michael R. Hamblin, a leading researcher in photomedicine, and Harry T. Whelan, a pioneer in the use of red light therapy in space medicine.

As we have seen, red light therapy has undergone remarkable development over the years. From Niels Ryberg Finsen's early studies to today's technological advances, a solid base of scientific knowledge and clinical applications has accumulated. Thanks to advances in technology and continuous research, red light therapy has evolved into an increasingly accessible and effective form of treatment for a variety of conditions and diseases. Modern red light devices offer precise and controlled light emission, allowing optimal therapy administration.

The scientific validation of red light therapy has been supported by numerous clinical and experimental studies. These studies have consistently shown beneficial effects on wound healing, pain reduction, improved muscle function, stimulation of hair growth, and other therapeutic benefits. In addition, research has been conducted on red light therapy in various medical areas, such as dermatology, physical therapy, neurology, and psychiatry.

Advances in red light therapy have also translated into its practical application. Currently, a wide variety of red light therapy devices are available on the market, ranging from desk lamps and light panels to portable devices for personal use. These devices allow patients to receive home treatment, which improves accessibility and comfort.

Red light therapy has also been integrated into various therapeutic approaches. It is used as a complementary therapy in combination with other treatments, such as physical therapy, medication, and cognitive-behavioral therapy. The combination of different therapeutic modalities can enhance the results and offer a comprehensive approach to health and well-being.

Red light therapy has undergone a significant evolution in its recognition and acceptance in the scientific and medical community. As more research and clinical studies have been conducted, an increasingly compelling evidence base has emerged that supports their efficacy in various medical conditions. This has led to its integration into medical and therapeutic practice in different specialties. Each of these aspects is addressed below:

Evolution of recognition: Initially, red light therapy was viewed with skepticism and considered as an alternative therapy. However, as more research and studies were conducted, positive and consistent results began to gain recognition in the scientific and medical community. This led to increased interest and acceptance of red light therapy as a valid therapeutic approach.

Clinical evidence: Clinical studies and systematic reviews have supported the efficacy of red light therapy in various medical conditions. For example, in the field of dermatology, research has been conducted that demonstrates its effectiveness in the treatment of acne, scars and skin aging. In the field of physical therapy, studies have been carried out that support its effectiveness in reducing pain, accelerating muscle recovery and improving physical function. These scientific findings have contributed to the recognition of red light therapy as a valid therapeutic approach.

Integration into medical and therapeutic practice: Red light therapy has been integrated into different medical and therapeutic specialties. For example, in physical therapy and rehabilitation, it is used to improve muscle recovery, reduce pain, and speed wound healing. In dermatology, it is used to treat skin conditions such as acne and skin aging. In addition, it has been used in psychiatry and neurology to treat mood disorders, such as depression and seasonal affective disorder. The integration of red light therapy into these specialties demonstrates its acceptance and recognition as a valid therapeutic approach.

Red light therapy has gained recognition and acceptance in the scientific and medical community as a solid evidence base has emerged that supports its efficacy in various medical conditions. Clinical studies and systematic reviews have supported its effectiveness in the treatment of dermatological conditions, mood disorders and musculoskeletal problems, among others. Moreover, its integration into medical and therapeutic practice in different specialties demonstrates its clinical relevance and status as a valid therapeutic approach.

The acceptance of red light therapy in the scientific and medical community has been further strengthened by rigorous clinical studies and systematic reviews. These studies have consistently shown the therapeutic benefits of red light therapy in various medical conditions.

For example, in the field of dermatology, clinical studies have demonstrated the efficacy of red light therapy in the treatment of skin diseases such as vitiligo, psoriasis and atopic dermatitis. These studies have provided convincing evidence that red light therapy can improve the appearance of the skin, reduce inflammation, and promote wound healing.

In the field of pain medicine, research has been conducted that supports the use of red light therapy in the relief of chronic pain, including back pain, arthritis, and sports injuries. These studies have shown that red light therapy can reduce inflammation, stimulate endorphin production, and improve blood circulation, which contributes to reducing pain and promoting healing.

Beyond clinical studies, systematic reviews and meta-analyzes have further consolidated evidence in support of red light therapy. These reviews have extensively examined existing studies and have provided a summary of the available evidence. They have concluded that red-light therapy is a promising and safe therapeutic option in several areas, supported by high-quality scientific evidence.

The integration of red light therapy into medical and therapeutic practice has been made possible by the growing scientific evidence and the development of more advanced and accessible red light technologies. Currently, portable, and home-use devices are available that enable patients to receive red-light therapy in the comfort of their homes, under the appropriate supervision of health care practitioners.

Red light therapy has gained recognition and acceptance in the scientific and medical community due to rigorous clinical studies, systematic reviews and meta-analyzes that support its efficacy in various medical conditions. Its integration into medical and therapeutic practice has provided patients with an additional therapeutic option supported by strong scientific evidence. As research continues and more technological advances are made, red light therapy is expected to remain a growing field in health and wellness.

Red light therapy has found applications in various fields of medicine, dermatology, and physiotherapy. Listed below are some of the current applications and possible areas of future application of red light therapy:

Sports medicine and physical therapy: Red light therapy is widely used in sports and physical therapy to speed up muscle recovery, reduce inflammation, and relieve pain in sports injuries. It has been shown to improve tissue healing and stimulate cell regeneration, which benefits athletes and people who are rehabilitating themselves from injury.

Dermatology and Skin Care: In dermatology, red light therapy has been used to treat skin conditions such as acne, skin aging, scars, and burns. It has been shown that red light stimulates collagen production, improves blood circulation, and promotes cell regeneration, resulting in healthier and rejuvenated skin.

Mood and sleep disorders: Red light therapy has shown potential benefits in treating mood disorders, such as depression and seasonal affective disorder. Exposure to red light can help regulate circadian rhythms, improve mood, and increase energy. Its effect on sleep disorders, such as insomnia and time lag, is also being investigated.

Neurology and Brain Health: Research is underway into the use of red light therapy in the treatment of neurological disorders, such as Alzheimer's disease, cognitive impairment, and traumatic brain injuries. Red light is thought to have neuroprotective effects and promote neuronal regeneration.

As for possible areas of future application, research is exploring the use of red light therapy in emerging fields such as oncology, gene therapy, and regenerative medicine. Its effects on cancer treatment, accelerating wound healing, tissue regeneration, and improving overall health are being investigated.

Emerging technologies related to red light therapy are impacting clinical practice. For example, more portable, flexible, and powerful devices are being developed to enable more precise and personalized therapy management. New wavelengths of light and color combinations are also being investigated to maximize therapeutic benefits.

POTENTIAL BENEFITS OF RED LIGHT THERAPY

Red light therapy has demonstrated several health and physical wellness benefits. Here are some of them and we will develop them later:

Improving wound healing and tissue regeneration: Red light penetrates deep layers of the skin and stimulates the production of ATP (adenosine triphosphate), which is the energy source of cells. This speeds up the wound healing process and promotes the regeneration of tissues, including skin, muscles, and bones. In addition, red light can help reduce scarring and improve the appearance of the wounds.

Pain relief and reduction of inflammation: Red light therapy has analgesic and anti-inflammatory properties. Red light helps block the pain pathways, resulting in a reduction in chronic, sharp pain. In addition, red light can reduce inflammation by inhibiting the release of certain inflammatory substances and promoting blood circulation, which helps deliver nutrients and oxygen to affected areas.

Stimulation of blood circulation: Red light improves microcirculation by dilating blood vessels and increasing local blood flow. This is beneficial for tissue oxygenation, metabolic waste disposal, and delivery of essential nutrients. Improved blood circulation can promote healing, relieve the feeling of tired legs, and contribute to overall cardiovascular health.

Increased collagen production and improved skin health: Red light stimulates fibroblasts in the skin to produce collagen, which is an essential protein for elasticity and skin health. An increase in collagen production can help reduce wrinkles and expression lines, improve skin texture, and promote a more youthful appearance. In addition, red light can also help reduce inflammation and improve skin conditions, such as acne and dermatitis.

Strengthening the immune system: Red light therapy can modulate the immune system, strengthening the body's immune response. Red light stimulates the activity of macrophages, which are cells responsible for phagocytosing and killing bacteria and other pathogens. It can also promote the proliferation of lymphocytes, which are key cells in the immune response. A strengthened immune system can help prevent infections and promote optimal health.

Emphasize that red light therapy is not a substitute for conventional medical treatments, but rather a complementary therapy. It is always advisable to consult a health professional before initiating any type of red light therapy, especially in cases of specific diseases or medical conditions.

Not only does red light therapy have physical benefits, but it can also have a positive impact on mental and emotional health. Here are some of the most prominent benefits:

Improving mood and reducing depression: Exposure to red light has been shown to be effective in improving mood and reducing symptoms of depression. Red light stimulates the release of endorphins and serotonin, neurotransmitters associated with well-being and happiness. In addition, red light therapy can regulate chemical imbalances in the brain and help stabilize mood.

Regulation of circadian rhythms and improvement of sleep: Exposure to red light can help regulate circadian rhythms, which are the body's natural cycles of sleep and wakefulness. Red light helps increase the production of melatonin, a hormone that regulates sleep. This can be beneficial for those suffering from sleep disorders, such as insomnia, and can also improve the overall quality of sleep.

Reducing stress and anxiety: Red light therapy can have relaxing and soothing effects on the body and mind. Exposure to red light helps reduce levels of cortisol, the stress hormone, and promotes the release of endorphins, which have analgesic and tranquilizing properties. This can help reduce stress and anxiety levels, providing a sense of calm and well-being.

Increased energy and vitality: Red light can stimulate metabolism and increase energy levels. Exposure to red light activates mitochondria in cells, resulting in increased production of ATP, the cellular energy source. This may be beneficial for those experiencing fatigue or lack of energy, as red light therapy can increase vitality levels and improve physical and mental performance.

Improved focus and concentration: Red light therapy can improve mental clarity, focus, and concentration. Red light stimulates brain activity and promotes blood circulation in the brain, which can help improve cognitive functions. This can be especially useful for students, professionals and anyone who wants to improve their intellectual performance.

As if there were not few benefits mentioned, red light therapy can also have other positive effects on mental and emotional health. Here are some additional areas where a beneficial impact has been observed:

Improved mood disorders: In addition to depression, red light therapy has shown benefits in other mood disorders, such as seasonal affective disorder (SAD) and bipolar disorder. Regular exposure to red light can help reduce symptoms associated with these disorders, such as changes in mood, lack of energy, and decreased motivation.

Reducing symptoms of anxiety disorders: Red light therapy may be beneficial in managing anxiety disorders, such as generalized anxiety disorder and posttraumatic stress disorder. Exposure to red light can promote relaxation, reduce muscle tension, and help control symptoms associated with anxiety, such as restlessness, agitation, and panic attacks.

Promoting emotional well-being: Red light therapy has been shown to have positive effects on overall emotional well-being. Exposure to red light can increase the production of hormones and neurotransmitters related to happiness and well-being, which can result in a general feeling of joy, optimism, and life satisfaction.

It is important to note that red light therapy is not a single treatment for severe mental and emotional disorders. However, it can be an effective adjunct when used as part of a comprehensive treatment approach that includes psychologic therapy, medication, and other therapeutic approaches.

Red light therapy has gained popularity in sports and physical performance due to its potential benefits for athletes and active people. Some of the most prominent benefits are described below:

Accelerating muscle recovery and reducing injury time: Red light therapy has been shown to be effective in speeding muscle recovery after vigorous exercise and in reducing injury time. Red light penetrates into muscle tissues and promotes blood circulation, which helps increase the supply of oxygen and nutrients to muscles as well as eliminate metabolic waste products. This can reduce inflammation, relieve muscle pain, and speed up the healing process of injuries.

Improved sports performance: Red light therapy can improve sports performance by increasing aerobic and anaerobic capacity. Exposure to red light stimulates energy production in cells, resulting in increased endurance and an increased ability to do high-intensity exercise. In addition, red light can improve mitochondrial function, which is essential for energy generation in the body. This can translate into better performance in sports activities and longer endurance time.

Increased muscle strength and endurance: Red light therapy may contribute to increased muscle strength and endurance. Red light stimulates protein synthesis and collagen production, which can aid in the construction and repair of muscle tissue. In addition, red light can increase the production of ATP, the cellular energy source, allowing for greater muscle contraction capacity and better endurance in exercise.

Reducing muscle fatigue: Red light therapy can help reduce muscle fatigue during and after exercise. Exposure to red light can speed the removal of lactic acid and other waste products accumulated in muscles during vigorous exercise. This can help reduce the feeling of fatigue and improve muscle recovery.

Red-light therapy may also help improve muscle flexibility and prevent injury. Red light stimulates the production of collagen, a protein essential for the health and elasticity of connective tissues. This can help maintain muscle and joint flexibility, which reduces the risk of stiffness-related injuries or lack of mobility.

Exposure to red light can have anti-inflammatory and analgesic effects on muscles. Red light enters the tissues and stimulates the release of nitric oxide, a compound that helps dilate blood vessels and improve blood flow. This can reduce inflammation and relieve muscle pain associated with intense exercise or injury.

Red light therapy improves blood circulation in muscle tissues, which helps increase the supply of oxygen and essential nutrients to muscles. This promotes better muscle recovery after exercise and favors the delivery of nutrients needed for protein synthesis and tissue repair.

Red light therapy can also have psychological benefits for athletes and active people. Exposure to red light can promote muscle and mental relaxation, thus reducing stress and the tension accumulated during training or competition. This can contribute to faster recovery and a sense of overall well-being.

Red light therapy has shown promising benefits in treating a variety of specific conditions. Some prominent examples are described below:

> Dermatological disorders: Red light therapy has been shown to be effective in the treatment of dermatological disorders such as acne, psoriasis, and vitiligo. Red light has anti-inflammatory properties and promotes skin healing. For acne, red light can reduce inflammation and the growth of acne-causing bacteria. In psoriasis, red light may help reduce redness and scaling of the skin. In vitiligo, red light can stimulate melanin production and improve skin pigmentation.

Sleep disorders: Red light therapy has been used to treat sleep disorders such as insomnia and time lag. Exposure to red light can help regulate circadian rhythms and promote better sleep quality. Red light stimulates the production of melatonin, a hormone that regulates sleep, which can facilitate sleep onset and improve sleep quality.

Neurodegenerative diseases: Preliminary research has suggested that red light therapy may have benefits in neurodegenerative diseases such as Alzheimer's and Parkinson's. Red light can stimulate mitochondrial function in brain cells and reduce inflammation, which can help protect and preserve cognitive function. However, more research is needed in this area to fully understand the effects of red light therapy on these diseases.

In addition, it is noteworthy that red light therapy can vary in terms of duration, intensity, and frequency depending on the specific condition and individual needs. Therefore, it is critical to work closely with trained health care practitioners specializing in red light therapy to obtain appropriate guidelines and protocols.

As research continues to advance in the field of red light therapy, more applications, and benefits in the treatment of various conditions are likely to be discovered. Advances in technology can also lead to the creation of more efficient and accessible devices, which will further expand the therapeutic potential of red light.

Red light therapy has also demonstrated significant benefits in the field of aesthetics and personal care.

Red light therapy can stimulate the production of collagen and elastin in the skin, two key proteins responsible for skin elasticity and firmness. This can help reduce the appearance of wrinkles and fine lines, providing a more youthful and smooth appearance.

Red light has anti-inflammatory and antioxidant properties that can help reduce spots, hyperpigmentation, and redness of the skin. In addition, it can help decrease the size of dilated pores, improving the overall texture of the skin and leaving it softer and more uniform.

Red light therapy can stimulate hair follicles and promote healthy hair growth. This can be beneficial both in the treatment of hair loss and in improving hair density and volume.

Red light can penetrate the deeper layers of the skin and help improve blood and lymphatic circulation, which can contribute to the reduction of localized cellulitis and fat. In addition, red light therapy can help stimulate cell metabolism, which can contribute to the elimination of toxins and the improvement of skin appearance in problem areas.

OTHER AESTHETIC APPLICATIONS

Red light can help improve the appearance of scars and stretch marks by promoting tissue regeneration and stimulating collagen production. This can lead to reduced visibility of scars and stretch marks, improving skin texture and tone.

Red light therapy has shown antibacterial and anti-inflammatory effects, which may be beneficial in the treatment of acne. Red light can help reduce inflammation, decrease sebum production, and promote healing of acne-related lesions.

Red light therapy has also been used in dentistry for the treatment of various oral conditions. It can help reduce gum inflammation, promote healing after tooth extractions or surgery, and treat conditions such as periodontitis and oral mucositis.

Red light can help improve blood circulation and oxygenation of facial tissues, which can lead to a more radiant and rejuvenated appearance. By stimulating the production of collagen and elastin, red light therapy can contribute to a firmer, toned, and revitalized facial appearance.

It is worth mentioning that red light therapy in the aesthetic and personal care field can be performed in specialized clinics using professional devices. There are also portable and home-use devices that allow you to perform red light treatments at home, although it is advisable to consult with a professional to obtain the appropriate indications and guidelines.

Red light therapy may also provide eye health benefits. Below are some of them:

> Improved eye health: Controlled exposure to red light can help promote overall eye health. Red light can stimulate blood circulation in eye tissues and improve the supply of nutrients and oxygen to the eyes, which can help maintain good eye health in the long term.

> Eye fatigue relief and reduction of dry eyes: Red light therapy can help relieve eye fatigue caused by long hours of work in front of computer screens, mobile devices, or other eye stressors. It can also help reduce dry eyes by stimulating the tear glands and increasing tear production.

> Stimulating tear production and improving dry eye syndrome: Dry eye syndrome is a common condition in which the eyes do not produce enough tears or tears are not of adequate quality to lubricate the eyes. Red light therapy may help stimulate the tear glands and improve tear production, thus relieving symptoms of dry eye syndrome.

> Improved night vision: Controlled exposure to red light may improve the ability to adapt visually in low-light conditions. This

may be especially beneficial for people who experience difficulties with night vision, such as problems driving at night or adapting to dimly lit environments.

It cannot be overlooked that red light therapy for eye health should be performed under the supervision of an eye health professional and using safe and appropriate devices. Each person may have different eye needs and conditions, so it is important to receive an individualized evaluation and an appropriate treatment plan.

Red light therapy has also shown benefits in healthy aging. Exposure to red light can stimulate energy production in cells and improve mitochondrial function. This can help slow cell aging and promote greater longevity.

Red light has antioxidant properties that can help neutralize free radicals and reduce oxidative stress in the body. This can help protect cells and tissues from damage caused by aging processes.

Red light therapy can stimulate brain activity and promote neuronal regeneration. This can have positive effects on cognitive function, memory, and prevention of neurodegenerative diseases such as Alzheimer's and Parkinson's.

Exposure to red light can improve vascular function and promote healthy blood circulation. This can help prevent cardiovascular disease and reduce the risk of conditions related to aging, such as hypertension and heart disease.

Red-light therapy can have bone health benefits by stimulating bone formation and improving bone density. This is especially relevant in aging since it is associated with an increased incidence of osteoporosis and risk of fractures. Red light can help strengthen bones and prevent age-related bone loss.

Exposure to red light can have positive effects on the body's metabolism. It has been observed that red light therapy can improve insulin sensitivity, regulate blood glucose levels, and promote fat burning. These benefits can help prevent metabolic diseases such as type 2 diabetes and obesity.

Red light can have anti-inflammatory properties and help reduce the chronic inflammation associated with aging. Chronic inflammation is a risk factor for many age-related diseases, such as heart disease, diabetes, and neurodegenerative diseases. Red light therapy can help modulate the body's inflammatory response and promote a state of balance.

Red light therapy can have a positive impact on the quality of life and general well-being of older people. The physical and mental benefits of red-light therapy, such as pain relief, improved sleep, reduced stress, and improved mood, may contribute to greater satisfaction and enjoyment of life in older age.

RED LIGHT THERAPY FUNDAMENTALS

LIGHT AS A THERAPY

Light is a fundamental element in our lives and has a significant impact on our health and well-being. Throughout history, we have recognized the power of light to influence various aspects of our existence, from regulating our circadian rhythms to affecting our mood and improving our physical health.

In recent years, light therapy has gained attention as an effective and non-invasive form of treatment in various health conditions. Light therapy is based on the idea that different wavelengths of light can penetrate biological tissues and trigger beneficial physiological and therapeutic responses.

Light therapy is based on a number of well-established scientific principles. One of them is the role of light in regulating our circadian rhythms. Our internal clock, known as the circadian rhythm, syncs primarily with natural daylight and dark night. Exposure to bright light during the day and absence of light at night help maintain a healthy circadian rhythm, which has an impact on our sleep quality, mood, and cognitive performance.

Another scientific foundation of light therapy is the effect of light on the production of neurotransmitters, such as serotonin and melatonin. These neurotransmitters play a crucial role in our mental and emotional health. Bright light, especially white light, and blue light, can stimulate the production of serotonin, known as the "happiness hormone", thus improving our mood and reducing the symptoms of depression and anxiety. On the other hand, exposure to dim, warm light in the hours before sleep can stimulate production of melatonin, the hormone responsible for regulating the sleep cycle, which helps us fall asleep more easily.

In addition, light therapy also relies on the effect of light in stimulating biological processes at the cellular level. Red and near-infrared light has the ability to penetrate deep into tissues and activate energy production in cellular mitochondria. This can improve blood circulation, accelerate wound healing, and promote tissue regeneration.

Light plays a key role in regulating our circadian rhythms, which are the internal cycles that control our sleep, wakefulness, hormones, and various physiological functions. Our circadian rhythm is mainly influenced by natural daylight and dark night.

When we are exposed to bright light during the day, especially blue light, a signal is sent to our brain to suppress the production of melatonin, a hormone that helps us fall asleep. This keeps us alert and awake during the day. On the other hand, when we are exposed to darkness or dim, warm light in the hours before sleep, melatonin production is stimulated, which helps us relax and prepare to sleep.

However, in modern society, we are exposed to sources of artificial light at night, such as screens of electronic devices, which emit blue light and can interfere with our circadian rhythms. This can lead to sleep disturbances, such as insomnia and time lag.

Light therapy has been shown to be effective in regulating circadian rhythms and sleep. Exposure to bright light and specifically to blue light during the day can help synchronize our internal clock and improve sleep quality. On the other hand, exposure to dim, warm light in the hours before sleep can facilitate melatonin production and promote more restful sleep.

Numerous studies support the efficacy of light therapy in sleep. For example, research has shown that exposure to bright light in the morning can reduce the symptoms of time lag and speed adaptation to new schedules. In addition, light therapy has been found to be beneficial for people who suffer from sleep disorders, such as insomnia, sleep phase delay syndrome, and seasonal affective disorder.

Light also has a major influence on our mental and emotional health. Exposure to bright light, especially natural daylight, can have positive effects on our mood and general well-being.

Lack of exposure to light during the winter months can lead to seasonal affective disorder (SAD), a type of seasonal depression that affects some people. Reduced sunlight and altered circadian rhythms are thought to trigger changes in levels of serotonin, a mood-related chemical in the brain. Light therapy, through exposure to bright light and specifically to white or blue light, has been shown to be effective in treating SAD, improving depressive symptoms, and increasing emotional well-being.

In addition to ART, light therapy has also shown benefits in other mood disorders, such as nonseasonal depression. Regular exposure to bright light can increase serotonin levels and reduce depressive symptoms. Improvement in anxiety and stress has also been observed, as light can help regulate the nervous system and promote a sense of calm and relaxation.

Light therapy is not only limited to mood disorders but can also be beneficial in low-energy, unmotivated situations. Exposure to bright light can increase vitality and energy, improving productivity and overall mood.

Scientific research supports the use of light therapy in mental health. Studies have shown that light therapy is effective in the treatment of SAD and non-seasonal depression, with results comparable to those of other therapeutic approaches, such as drug therapy or cognitive-behavioral therapy. In addition, testimonials from individuals who have used light therapy highlight a significant improvement in their mood, energy levels and overall well-being.

Light not only influences our mood and mental health, but also has a significant impact on our physical health and general well-being. Proper exposure to light can trigger a number of beneficial biological responses in our body.

The physical benefits associated with light exposure could be summarized schematically in:

Regulating circadian rhythms: Regular daytime exposure to natural light helps regulate our circadian rhythms, which are the internal biological cycles that control various physiological functions, such as sleep, body temperature, and metabolism.

Improving vitamin D: Sunlight is an important source of vitamin D, which is essential for bone health and the immune system. Exposure to sunlight helps the body make vitamin D naturally.

Stimulating energy and alertness: Bright light, especially white or blue light, can increase energy and mental alertness, contributing to increased productivity and physical performance.

In conclusion, light plays a fundamental role in our health and well-being, both physically and mentally. The mechanisms of action of light in the human body are diverse and complex, ranging from regulating circadian rhythms to modulating neurotransmitters and hormones.

Light therapy has proven to be an effective and safe therapeutic option in a wide range of medical and wellness conditions. Scientific studies support its effectiveness in sleep disorders, mood disorders, dermatologic conditions, sports injuries, and more. Testimonials from people who have experienced significant benefits also support its use.

ELECTROMAGNETIC SPECTRUM AND VISIBLE LIGHT

The electromagnetic spectrum is a representation of all possible frequencies and wavelengths of electromagnetic waves. These waves are a form of energy that spreads through space and span a wide range of frequencies, from highest to lowest.

The electromagnetic spectrum consists of different regions, each with distinct characteristics and properties. These regions include gamma radiation, x-rays, ultraviolet rays, visible light, microwaves, and radio waves.

Gamma radiation: This region of the electromagnetic spectrum has the highest frequencies and shortest wavelengths. Gamma radiation is used in nuclear medicine and in industrial applications.

X-rays: X-rays have lower frequencies and longer wavelengths than gamma radiation. They are used in medicine to image the inside of the body and in security applications such as airport baggage screening.

Ultraviolet rays: Ultraviolet rays have lower frequencies and longer wavelengths than X-rays. They are divided into three categories: UV-A, UV-B and UV-C. UV-C has the shortest wavelength and is used in disinfection applications.

Visible light: Visible light is the part of the electromagnetic spectrum that we can perceive with our eyes. It comprises a range of colors from violet to red. Visible light is responsible for vision and plays a significant role in color perception.

Microwaves: Microwaves have lower frequencies and longer wavelengths than visible light. They are used in applications such as wireless communication and food heating.

Radio waves: Radio waves have the lowest frequencies and the longest wavelengths in the electromagnetic spectrum. They are used for radio, television, mobile telephony, and wireless communications in general.

Each region of the electromagnetic spectrum has specific applications and properties. Visible light is particularly relevant in light therapy, as our ability to perceive and respond to visible light has a significant impact on our health and well-being.

Visible light is the portion of the electromagnetic spectrum that is perceptible to the human eye. It is located between the regions of ultraviolet (UV) and infrared (IR) radiation. Unlike other forms of electromagnetic radiation, such as X-rays or microwaves, visible light is what we can see and experience directly.

Visible light is composed of a variety of colors ranging from violet to red. These colors are what we see when white light breaks down at different wavelengths. The visible spectrum colors, in ascending order of wavelength, are as follows:

Violet: It is the color with the shortest wavelength and highest energy in the visible spectrum. It is located near the ultraviolet end.

Blue: It has a slightly longer wavelength than violet, but it is still a short wavelength compared to other colors.

Green: The color of the middle of the visible spectrum and has an intermediate wavelength.

Yellow: It has a wavelength slightly longer than green.

Orange: It has a longer wavelength than yellow.

Red: It is the color with the longest wavelength and lowest energy in the visible spectrum. It is located near the infrared end.

The wavelength of visible light ranges from about 400 nanometers (nm) at the violet end to about 700 nm at the red end. The frequency of visible light is inversely related to wavelength, which means that colors with shorter wavelengths have higher frequencies and vice versa.

The relationship between wavelength and color is based on how the human eye perceives light. Each visible color has a characteristic wavelength and frequency, and when these colors are combined in different proportions, we perceive a wide range of tones and shades in the world around us.

In light therapy, distinct colors of visible light are used for different therapeutic purposes, taking advantage of the specific properties of each color in relation to the biological response of the human body.

Visible light has several properties and characteristics that make it unique and fundamental for our visual perception and the study of its interaction with objects. Here are some of these properties:

Reflection: Visible light can be reflected on the surface of objects. When light hits an object, some of it is absorbed and some of it is reflected. The reflected light is captured by our eyes, allowing us to see the object. How light is reflected depends on the texture, color, and composition of the object.

Refraction: Refraction occurs when visible light passes from one medium to another with different density, as when light passes from air to water or from air to glass. As the medium changes, the speed of the light changes, causing a change in its direction. This is what allows us to see the deviation of light as it passes through a lens or a prism.

Scattering: Scattering is a phenomenon in which visible light is separated into its components of different colors due to its different wavelength. This happens, for example, when white light passes through a prism and breaks down into a spectrum of colors. Dispersion is responsible for rainbow formation and other related optical phenomena.

Visible light is perceived by the human eye because of the presence of light-sensitive cells in the retina called cones and rods. Cones are responsible for color vision and work best in bright light conditions, while rods are more sensitive to dim light and allow us to see in black and white.

When visible light reaches our eyes, it passes through the cornea and lens, which are transparent structures that focus light on the retina. There, the photoreceptors convert light into electrical signals that are transmitted to the brain through the optic nerve. The brain interprets these electrical signals as visual images.

The interaction of visible light with objects depends on factors such as absorption, reflection, and transmission. Some objects selectively absorb certain light colors, giving them a characteristic color. Other objects reflect light more evenly, resulting in a more neutral appearance. In addition, some objects can transmit light through them, allowing their passage and generating transparency effects.

Visible light plays a fundamental role in our daily lives and in the functioning of organisms. Here are some of the essential functions of visible light:

Vision: The most obvious function of visible light is to allow us to see the world around us. Our visual system is able to detect different wavelengths of visible light and transform them into visual images in the brain. Thanks to visible light, we can perceive shapes, colors, textures, and depth in our environment.

Color perception: Visible light is composed of a range of colors from violet to red. Our eyes and our brains are able to interpret different wavelengths of light as different colors. This ability allows us to appreciate and distinguish a wide variety of shades and nuances in the world around us.

Regulation of circadian rhythms: Visible light also plays a crucial role in regulating our circadian rhythms, which are the natural cycles of activity and rest that occur over a period of approximately 24 hours. Exposure to visible light, especially bright blue light, helps synchronize our circadian rhythms and maintain a proper sleep-wake cycle. This influences our energy, mood, cognitive performance and many other aspects of our health and well-being.

In addition to these key functions, visible light also has effects on other aspects of the biology and functioning of organisms. For example, in plants, visible light is essential for photosynthesis, the process by which plants convert light energy into chemical energy for their growth and development. It has also been discovered that visible light can influence the production of hormones and neurotransmitters in the human body, which has an impact on health and mood.

Visible light plays a significant role in various light therapy modalities, such as red light therapy and blue light therapy. These therapies use different wavelengths of visible light to achieve specific therapeutic effects in the human body. These modalities and how wavelength and intensity of visible light influence their effects are briefly described below:

Red light therapy: Red light therapy uses wavelengths of light in the visible range near the red, usually around 630-660 nanometers. This specific wavelength of red light has been shown to have beneficial effects on health and well-being. Red light is believed to penetrate deep into the body's tissues, stimulating cell energy production and promoting cell regeneration and repair. Red light has also been shown to help reduce inflammation, relieve pain, improve blood circulation, and stimulate collagen production, among other benefits.

Blue Light Therapy: On the other hand, blue light therapy uses wavelengths of light in the visible range near the blue, typically around 450-470 nanometers. Blue light has been associated with stimulating and regulating effects on circadian rhythms. Exposure to bright blue light during the day can help increase energy, improve alertness, and regulate sleep-wake rhythms. However, exposure to blue light at night, especially from electronic devices, can interfere with sleep quality because of its impact on the production of melatonin, a hormone that regulates sleep.

The wavelength and intensity of visible light are key factors in light therapy, as they determine the specific effects on the human body. Each wavelength has different penetration and absorption into tissues, which influences how deep it can reach and what effects it can trigger. In addition, the intensity of light, i.e., the amount of light energy reaching a specific surface, can also be adjusted to achieve the desired effect.

MECHANISMS OF ACTION OF RED LIGHT

Red light is a part of the electromagnetic spectrum found in the region of longer wavelengths and low energy. This light, with a wavelength of approximately 620 to 700 nanometers, is perceptible to the human eye and has been found to have beneficial therapeutic effects in various fields of health and well-being.

Understanding the mechanisms of action of red light is essential to maximize its therapeutic benefits. Although research in this field is still ongoing, it has been observed that red light interacts with the cells and tissues of the body, triggering a series of biochemical and physiological responses.

One of the main mechanisms of action of red light is related to the stimulation of adenosine triphosphate (ATP) production in mitochondria, the structures responsible for generating energy in cells. Red light appears to increase the efficiency of ATP production, providing additional energy for cellular functions and promoting tissue regeneration and repair.

In addition, red light has been shown to have anti-inflammatory and analgesic properties. By interacting with tissues, red light can reduce inflammation and relieve pain. This effect is partly attributed to the release of nitric oxide, a chemical which improves blood circulation and has analgesic properties.

Another important mechanism of action of red light is its ability to stimulate the production of collagen, a protein key in the health of the skin, tendons, and bones. Red light can increase collagen synthesis, which helps improve skin elasticity and firmness as well as speed wound healing.

It has been observed that red light can regulate circadian rhythms and improve sleep. Exposure to red light may influence the production of melatonin, a hormone that regulates sleep and wake cycles. Red light promotes melatonin production, which helps regulate circadian rhythms and contributes to healthy sleep.

Red light is a part of the electromagnetic spectrum found in the region of longer wavelengths and low energy. This light, with a wavelength of approximately 620 to 700 nanometers, is perceptible to the human eye and has been found to have beneficial therapeutic effects in various fields of health and well-being.

Understanding the mechanisms of action of red light is essential to maximize its therapeutic benefits. Although research in this field is still ongoing, it has been observed that red light interacts with the cells and tissues of the body, triggering a series of biochemical and physiological responses.

One of the main mechanisms of action of red light is related to the stimulation of adenosine triphosphate (ATP) production in mitochondria, the structures responsible for generating energy in cells. Red light appears to increase the efficiency of ATP production, providing additional energy for cellular functions and promoting tissue regeneration and repair.

It has also been observed that red light has anti-inflammatory and analgesic properties. By interacting with tissues, red light can reduce inflammation and relieve pain. This effect is partly attributed to the release of nitric oxide, a chemical which improves blood circulation and has analgesic properties.

Another important mechanism of action of red light is its ability to stimulate the production of collagen, a protein key in the health of the skin, tendons, and bones. Red light can increase collagen synthesis, which helps improve skin elasticity and firmness as well as speed wound healing.

In addition, it has been observed that red light can regulate circadian rhythms and improve sleep. Exposure to red light may influence the production of melatonin, a hormone that regulates sleep and wake cycles. Red light promotes melatonin production, which helps regulate circadian rhythms and contributes to healthy sleep.

Red light has been shown to have anti-inflammatory and analgesic properties, making it an effective therapy to reduce inflammation and relieve pain in different tissues and organs of the body.

The ability of red light to reduce inflammation is partly due to its ability to stimulate the release of nitric oxide (NO) into cells. Nitric oxide is a signaling molecule that plays a significant role in the regulation of vascular function and inflammatory response. Red light induces the production of nitric oxide in cells, which improves blood circulation and promotes vasodilation. As a result, blood flow to the affected area increases, helping to reduce inflammation by bringing nutrients and oxygen to damaged tissues and removing waste products.

Apart from its anti-inflammatory action, red light also has analgesic properties that can relieve pain. Nitric oxide released in response to red light has vasodilatory and pain-modulating effects. By increasing blood flow and improving tissue oxygenation, red light can relieve the sensation of pain. In addition, red light has been shown to reduce the sensitivity of pain receptors on peripheral nerves, which decreases the transmission of pain signals to the central nervous system.

The anti-inflammatory and analgesic action of red light may be beneficial in a variety of conditions and lesions. It has been used successfully to reduce inflammation and pain in conditions such as arthritis, muscle injuries, neuropathies, fibromyalgia, and chronic inflammatory disorders. In addition, red light therapy has proven to be a safe and effective alternative to traditional analgesic drugs, as it does not present significant side effects or risk of addiction.

Red light has been shown to be effective in stimulating the production of collagen, a protein essential for health and tissue regeneration in the human body. Collagen is a key structural component present in the skin, tendons, bones, and other connective tissues, and plays a fundamental role in its strength, elasticity, and regenerative capacity.

When red light penetrates the skin and tissues, it activates cells called fibroblasts, which are responsible for collagen production. Red light stimulates fibroblasts to increase collagen synthesis, which in turn improves tissue structure and quality. In addition, red light can also increase the activity of the enzymes responsible for collagen formation, thereby speeding up their production and promoting faster regeneration of damaged or injured tissues.

Stimulating collagen production by using red light has several benefits. On the skin, it can improve elasticity, firmness, and overall appearance, which is especially beneficial in the treatment of wrinkles, fine lines, and scars. In tendons and muscle tissues, collagen production can help strengthen and repair damaged structures, improving function and reducing the risk of recurring injuries. In addition, in bone, collagen synthesis promoted by red light may contribute to increased bone density and improved fracture healing.

Red light also accelerates wound healing by stimulating tissue regeneration. By increasing collagen production, red light improves the formation of new blood vessels and granulation tissue at the wound site, accelerating the healing process. In addition, red light has antimicrobial properties, which helps prevent wound infections and promotes faster and uncomplicated healing.

Red light also plays a key role in regulating circadian rhythms and promoting healthy sleep. Circadian rhythms are the internal biological cycles that regulate our sleep and wake patterns as well as other physiological and metabolic functions. These rhythms are influenced by exposure to light, especially at certain wavelengths, such as red light.

Red light has a lower ability to suppress melatonin production compared to other wavelengths, such as blue light. Melatonin is a naturally occurring hormone in the body and plays a crucial role in regulating sleep. It is secreted in greater quantities in the dark, helping to induce sleep and maintain a healthy sleep rhythm.

When we are exposed to red light at night, especially before bedtime, melatonin production is less affected compared to exposure to other wavelengths of light. This is beneficial for the regulation of circadian rhythms, as it allows melatonin levels to increase appropriately, preparing the body for sleep.

Red light therapy can be used strategically to regulate circadian rhythms and improve sleep. Exposure to red light in the morning or during the day can help synchronize the circadian rhythm, promoting increased alertness and wakefulness during the day. On the other hand, limiting exposure to blue light and opting for red light in the hours before sleep can help reduce melatonin suppression and facilitate sleep onset.

In addition to its biochemical and regenerative effects, red light also exhibits antioxidant properties that can help protect cells against oxidative stress and damage caused by free radicals. Free radicals are highly reactive molecules that are naturally generated in the body as a result of normal metabolic processes and exposure to environmental factors, such as ultraviolet radiation, pollution, and stress.

Oxidative stress occurs when there is an imbalance between free radical production and the body's antioxidant defenses. Free radicals can damage cells and cell structures, contributing to aging, inflammation, and various disorders.

Red light has been shown to have antioxidant effects by stimulating the production of endogenous antioxidant enzymes, such as superoxide dismutase (SOD) and catalase. These enzymes play a crucial role in neutralizing free radicals and protecting cells against oxidative stress.

By exposing cells and tissues to red light, an increase in the activity of these antioxidant enzymes occurs, leading to an increased ability to neutralize free radicals and reduce oxidative stress. This, in turn, can help prevent cell damage, promote cell health, and contribute to healthier aging.

Apart from its antioxidant action, red light can also protect cells against damage caused by damaging environmental factors, such as ultraviolet radiation and contaminants. Exposure to red light can help mitigate the negative effects of ultraviolet radiation by increasing the activity of DNA repair enzymes and promoting cell regeneration.

Red light can also counteract oxidative stress caused by exposure to environmental pollutants and toxins. By stimulating the body's antioxidant defenses, red light can help protect cells and tissues from the harmful effects of pollutants, thereby reducing the risk of diseases related to environmental toxicity.

BIOLOGICAL EFFECTS OF RED LIGHT THERAPY

Red light causes biological effects on our body. Red light therapy stimulates the activity of mitochondria, the cellular structures responsible for energy production in the form of ATP. By increasing ATP production, red light therapy provides cells with the energy needed to perform their vital functions optimally, contributing to cell health and performance.

It also improves blood circulation by dilating blood vessels and increasing blood flow through them. This facilitates the delivery of oxygen and nutrients to tissues, as well as the disposal of metabolic wastes and toxins. Better blood circulation promotes cardiovascular health and the proper functioning of body systems.

Among others, it stimulates tissue regeneration and repair by increasing cell activity and protein synthesis. It stimulates healthy cell proliferation, new blood vessel formation and collagen synthesis, contributing to wound healing, reducing inflammation, and improving tissue health.

And finally, among the most relevant, influence on the production of hormones and neurotransmitters in the body. For example, it can stimulate the production of endorphins, known as the "happiness hormones," which have analgesic and antidepressant effects. In addition, it can regulate the production of melatonin, a key hormone in regulating circadian rhythms and sleep.

APPLICATIONS OF RED LIGHT

If we ask how long we should use red light therapy to see benefits in different areas, the answer varies depending on several factors: the device used, the duration and frequency of the sessions, and the specific health issues being treated. Some people notice a reduction in pain and inflammation after just one session of red light therapy. In my personal experience, it takes longer to feel the benefits in my practice. I have also observed that these devices accelerate wound healing and aid in post-workout recovery, generally after a few sessions.

On the other hand, for something like hair regeneration, red light therapy can take much longer, possibly months or even years of regular use before seeing results. As I mentioned, it depends on many variables, the most important being what is meant by "benefits."

The type of device used also influences the results. Clinical lasers usually offer faster results but only in small areas of the body and with a higher risk of side effects. On the other hand, an LED light device has no known side effects, making achieving results much safer.

The size of the device also affects the results. If you are looking to increase your energy level, a larger lamp will provide faster results. To improve collagen in the face or other specific areas, a smaller lamp is sufficient.

Let us see how we can apply red light to our bodies.

RED LIGHT THERAPY IN MOOD DISORDERS

The administration of red light therapy in the treatment of mood disorders may vary according to individual needs and the severity of symptoms. Although it is important to consult a health care practitioner before starting treatment, here are some general guidelines about recommended treatment protocols:

1-   Duration of exposure:

The duration of exposure to red light may vary, but generally it is recommended to start with sessions of 15 to 30 minutes a day.

Over time, duration may gradually increase based on individual response and health care practitioner recommendations.

2-   Light intensity:

The intensity of red light used in therapy can vary and is measured in lux (unit of illuminance).

It is suggested to use moderate to high intensity light, with a typical intensity ranging from 5,000 to 10,000 lux.

3-   Treatment schedule:

Red light therapy is usually done daily, preferably at the same time each day.

Morning light therapy is recommended because it can help regulate circadian rhythms and improve mood during the day.

The total duration of the treatment program may vary, but it is often recommended to perform therapy over several weeks or months for optimal results.

Note that these guidelines are general and can be adjusted based on individual needs and recommendations by the health care practitioner. In addition, red light therapy is usually combined with other therapeutic approaches, such as psychotherapy and drug use, depending on the severity and specific type of mood disorder.

Red light therapy has shown potential benefits in treating mood disorders and reducing depressive symptoms. Some of the important benefits and considerations associated with this form of treatment are listed below:

Improved mood: Regular exposure to red light can help improve mood and reduce depressive symptoms. Red light is thought to stimulate the release of neurotransmitters, such as serotonin, which are associated with mood regulation.

Increased energy: Red light therapy can increase energy levels and combat fatigue and lack of motivation, common symptoms in mood disorders. This can contribute to a greater sense of vitality and general well-being.

Circadian Rhythm Regulation: Red light can help regulate circadian rhythms, which are the natural cycles of the body that control wakefulness and sleep. By regulating circadian rhythms, red light therapy can improve sleep quality and promote a more regular sleep pattern.

Red light therapy should not be considered as a substitute for other recommended treatments for mood disorders, such as psychotherapy or medication. It can be used as a complementary tool in the overall treatment plan under the supervision of a health care practitioner.

Maria, a 35-year-old woman diagnosed with major depressive disorder, participated in a clinical study investigating the effects of red light therapy on mood. During treatment, you were given daily exposure to red light for 30 minutes for several weeks. At the end of the study, a significant improvement in Maria's depressive symptoms was observed, with a reduction in sadness, fatigue, and lack of energy.

Juan, a 45-year-old man who had experienced recurrent episodes of depression, decided to try red light therapy as part of his treatment plan. After using red light therapy regularly for several weeks, John reported a noticeable improvement in his mood. He felt more energetic, motivated and with a more positive attitude towards life. In addition, he noticed a reduction in physical symptoms associated with depression, such as sleep disturbances and loss of appetite.

These case studies and testimonials illustrate how red light therapy may be beneficial in the treatment of mood disorders. However, it is important to note that results may vary from person to person and that red light therapy should be used under the supervision of a health care practitioner.

RED LIGHT THERAPY IN SLEEP DISORDERS

Sleep disorders are conditions that affect the quality, duration, and regularity of sleep. These disorders can have a significant impact on a person's overall health and well-being. Sleep is essential for optimal functioning of the body and mind, and sleep disorders can interfere with natural sleep patterns, leading to physical, mental, and emotional health problems.

Among the most common sleep disorders are:

Insomnia: It is characterized by difficulty falling asleep, staying asleep, or waking up too early. People with insomnia often experience fatigue, lack of energy, and difficulty concentrating during the day.

Sleep apnea: Occurs when breathing is repeatedly interrupted during sleep due to a blockage in the airways. This can cause loud snoring and pauses in breathing, which interrupts sleep and can lead to daytime sleepiness and long-term health problems.

Circadian rhythm sleep disorder: Involves a mismatch between the natural rhythm of sleep and social or work programming. People with this disorder may have difficulty falling asleep at the desired time and experience excessive daytime sleepiness.

These sleep disorders not only affect people's quality of life but can also contribute to more serious health problems, such as cardiovascular disease, obesity, diabetes, and mood disorders.

Addressing these sleep disorders adequately and effectively is critical to restoring healthy sleep and improving quality of life. Red light therapy has emerged as a promising therapeutic option in the treatment of sleep disorders, as it can positively influence circadian rhythms and promote better sleep regulation. In the following points, we will explore how red light therapy can be used in the treatment of these specific disorders, providing a safe and effective option to improve the quality and quantity of sleep.

Red light therapy can be given in several ways to treat sleep disorders. Here are some of the most common methods:

Red light lamps: Red light lamps emit a specific wavelength light within the red range. These lamps are usually compact and portable, allowing use in different environments, such as the bedroom. They can be placed near the rest area or in a strategic position to be exposed to red light for the recommended time.

Red light panels: Red light panels consist of a larger surface that emits red light. These panels are typically more powerful than lamps and can cover a wider area. They can be wall mounted or placed on a stand for more comfortable and extended exposure.

Red light glasses: Red light glasses are another method of administering light therapy. These special glasses are designed to block other wavelengths of light and allow only red light transmission. By wearing the glasses, you can filter the ambient light and focus the exposure directly on the eyes.

Each of these methods of administration has its specific advantages and considerations. The choice of method will depend on individual preferences and the recommendations of the health care practitioner.

It is important to mention that red light therapy for sleep disorders is usually given in the morning or early in the day, since exposure to red light at night can interfere with the natural regulation of sleep.

When considering the option of red light devices, it is essential to look for quality products and certificates that meet safety and efficacy standards.

Red light therapy offers a promising, noninvasive way to address sleep disorders and improve the quality of rest. In the following points, we will explore in more detail the benefits and effectiveness of red light therapy in the treatment of specific sleep disorders.

The potential benefits of red light therapy in regulating circadian rhythms and improving sleep:

Establishing regular sleep patterns: Exposure to red light can help regulate circadian rhythms, which are the biological cycles that regulate sleep and wakefulness. By being exposed to red light at specific times of day, it can help synchronize the body's internal clock and establish more regular sleep patterns. This is especially beneficial for people who have difficulty falling asleep or who experience sleep disturbances related to the dysregulation of circadian rhythms.

Reducing difficulty falling asleep: Exposure to red light before bedtime can help reduce difficulty falling asleep. Red light has a soothing, calming effect, which can ease the transition to sleep. In addition, red light helps suppress the production of melatonin, a hormone that regulates sleep and is usually released in greater amounts in response to darkness. By modulating melatonin production with red light, the ability to fall asleep can be improved more quickly and effectively.

Improving sleep quality: Red light therapy can improve sleep quality by promoting deeper, more restful sleep. Exposure to red light during the day helps regulate circadian rhythms, which in turn facilitates consolidation of nighttime sleep. Quality sleep is associated with a greater sense of rest, increased energy during the day, and improved cognitive and emotional functioning.

Note that red light therapy for regulation of circadian rhythms and improvement of sleep is usually given in the morning or early in the day, avoiding exposure to red light near bedtime, as this can interfere with the body's ability to produce melatonin and prepare for rest.

Carlos, 50, suffered from circadian rhythm sleep disorder due to his night work. This caused him difficulty sleeping during the day and maintaining a regular sleep schedule. After consultation with a sleep disorder specialist, it was recommended to use a red light therapy light during your night shift. The red light simulated the natural sunlight and helped regulate his circadian rhythm. After a few weeks of using red light therapy during his night shift, Carlos experienced a noticeable improvement in his ability to fall asleep during the day and maintain a more regular sleep schedule. He felt more energetic and alert during his work shifts.

RED LIGHT THERAPY IN PAIN MANAGEMENT

Red light therapy has been shown to be beneficial in relieving muscle and joint pain. This is mostly due to:

Red light can penetrate muscle and joint tissues.

It stimulates local blood circulation, which helps provide nutrients and oxygen to damaged tissues.

It reduces inflammation in the muscles and joints, thus relieving pain and improving mobility.

It also provides additional benefits, such as muscle relaxation and reduced stiffness.

It has also been shown to be effective in the treatment of chronic conditions such as fibromyalgia, arthritis and in the relief of postoperative pain and in the recovery of injuries.

Pedro's testimony: "For years, I suffered from chronic pains in my back due to an injury at work. After trying different treatment approaches, I decided to try red light therapy. It was amazing how the pain started to subside after just a few sessions. Now I can enjoy a better quality of life and do activities that were previously impossible. Red light therapy has been a game changer for me."

RED LIGHT APPLED IN SKIN HEALTH

The skin, as the largest organ of the human body, plays a fundamental role in our health and well-being. It is our first line of defense against external elements and acts as a protective barrier that helps keep us safe from infections, injuries, and excessive water loss.

In addition to its protective function, the skin also has a significant impact on our appearance and self-esteem. Healthy, radiant skin makes us look and feel good, while skin problems can affect our confidence and quality of life.

Therefore, it is crucial to take proper care of our skin to keep it healthy and in its best condition. This involves adopting daily care habits, such as cleaning it properly, moisturizing it, protecting it from the sun and using products suitable for our skin type. It also means seeking treatments and therapies that can help us address specific skin problems and improve your overall appearance.

In this context, red light therapy has become a popular and promising skin care option. This noninvasive therapy uses specific wavelengths of red light to stimulate beneficial responses in the skin and promote its health and vitality. Throughout this chapter, we will explore in detail the benefits and application of red light therapy in skin care, as well as the important considerations to consider.

Red light therapy is a safe, non-invasive approach that uses specific wavelengths of red light to improve the health and appearance of the skin. Unlike more aggressive treatments, such as surgical procedures or laser treatments, red light therapy causes no damage or injury to the skin, making it an attractive option for many people.

The red light used in this therapy has a unique ability to penetrate the surface layers of the skin safely. Although it does not penetrate as deeply as other wavelengths, such as infrared light, it has the ability to activate beneficial biological responses in skin cells.

When red light reaches the skin, it is absorbed by cells and tissues. Red light energy is converted into cellular energy, stimulating the production of adenosine triphosphate (ATP) in the mitochondria, which is the source of energy needed for vital cellular functions. This increase in ATP production boosts cellular activity and promotes better skin function.

In addition, red light also has the ability to stimulate blood circulation in the skin. By increasing vasodilation, blood flow to the skin is improved, resulting in increased delivery of oxygen and nutrients to skin cells. This not only promotes healthier skin, but can also speed up wound healing and regeneration of damaged tissue.

1-   Stimulation of collagen production:

Red light is known for its ability to stimulate collagen production in the skin, resulting in improved skin elasticity and firmness. Collagen is a key protein in the structure of the skin and is responsible for providing strength and support. As we age, collagen production decreases, which can lead to the appearance of wrinkles and sagging.

Red light therapy works effectively by stimulating fibroblasts, cells in the skin dermis that are responsible for producing collagen. When exposed to red light, fibroblasts increase their activity and synthesize more collagen. This helps to strengthen the collagen matrix in the skin, improving its structure and texture.

Stimulating collagen production by using red light therapy has several skin benefits. It helps reduce the appearance of fine lines and wrinkles, as the skin becomes firmer and tighter. In addition, collagen also contributes to skin hydration, which helps keep the skin soft and radiant.

2-   Reduction of wrinkles and expression lines:

Red light therapy can be effective in reducing visible signs of aging, such as wrinkles and fine lines. When red light penetrates the skin, it stimulates the production of collagen and elastin, which are essential components to maintain the elasticity and flexibility of the skin.

Elastin is a protein that allows the skin to regain its shape after being stretched or contracted. Over time and due to factors such as sun exposure and collagen loss, elastin becomes weaker, resulting in the formation of wrinkles and expression lines. Red light therapy helps promote elastin production, which can improve skin elasticity and reduce the appearance of wrinkles.

In addition, red light can also stimulate cell renewal and the production of hyaluronic acid, a substance that retains moisture in the skin, helping to moisturize it and soften expression lines.

3-		Improving skin texture and tone:

Red light therapy can help improve the appearance of the skin by addressing different problems, such as spots, enlarged pores, and redness. Red light penetrates the skin's surface layers, stimulating blood circulation and promoting cell regeneration.

For spots, red light can help reduce the excess production of melanin, the pigment responsible for skin coloration. By regulating the activity of melanocytes, the cells that produce melanin, red light therapy can attenuate spots and improve overall skin tone, providing a more uniform appearance.

Red light may also have a beneficial effect on dilated pores. By stimulating blood circulation and promoting cell renewal, red light therapy can help reduce pore size and improve skin texture. In addition, by increasing collagen production, red light can strengthen the structure of the skin and make the pores appear less visible.

As for redness, red light therapy has anti-inflammatory properties that can help reduce skin irritation and inflammation. This may be beneficial for people with facial flushing, such as those with rosacea. Red light can soothe the skin and reduce the appearance of redness, promoting a more even skin tone.

4-		Treatment of acne:

Red light therapy has also been shown to be effective in the treatment of acne. Red light has antibacterial properties that can help eliminate acne-causing bacteria, such as Propionibacterium acnes. In addition, red light has anti-inflammatory properties that can reduce acne-associated inflammation and promote skin healing.

When applied directly to areas affected by acne, red light therapy can penetrate the skin and stimulate the production of adenosine triphosphate (ATP) in the mitochondria of cells. This provides additional energy to the cells, which speeds up the skin's repair and regeneration processes.

In addition, red light therapy can help reduce sebum production, excess fat that contributes to pore clogging, and comedone formation. By regulating the activity of the sebaceous glands, red light can decrease the appearance of new acne outbreaks.

Before initiating any treatment of red light therapy in skin care, it is important to seek professional guidance from a dermatologist. A dermatologist will be able to evaluate the skin condition and determine if red light therapy is suitable for each individual, as well as provide personalized recommendations.

It is essential to follow the instructions provided by the manufacturer of the red light therapy device. Each device may have specific recommendations regarding session duration, distance to place the device from the skin, and frequency of use. Also, regular follow-up with a health care practitioner is important to evaluate results and adjust treatment if necessary. During red light therapy, it is necessary to protect the eyes to avoid possible damage. Red light can be strong and potentially harmful to the eyes. It is recommended to wear protective goggles specifically designed to block red light during therapy sessions. These glasses will help protect your eyes and ensure a safe experience.

Some people may be more sensitive to light and may experience irritation or discomfort during red light therapy. If any significant discomfort or irritation occurs, treatment should be discontinued and a health care professional consulted.

Red light therapy may complement other skin care treatments, such as topical products or cosmetic procedures. However, it is important to tell a health care practitioner about any other treatments being done to make sure there are no negative interactions.

Other therapeutic uses of red light

Red light therapy has been shown to be effective in treating skin disorders such as psoriasis and eczema. Red light penetrates the surface layers of the skin, stimulating beneficial biological responses that help reduce the symptoms of these conditions.

Psoriasis is a chronic skin condition characterized by the appearance of scaly patches, redness, and itching. Red light therapy, also known as phototherapy therapy therapy, has been shown to be effective in reducing inflammation and peeling of the skin in patients with psoriasis. Controlled exposure to red light can decrease excessive proliferation of skin cells and regulate the immune system, leading to an improvement in symptoms.

Eczema, also known as atopic dermatitis, is a skin condition characterized by redness, itching and inflammation. Red light therapy may help relieve eczema symptoms by reducing skin inflammation and irritation. Red light promotes blood circulation and improves skin barrier function, which can decrease dryness and itching.

The benefits of red light therapy in the treatment of skin disorders such as psoriašis and eczema include reducing inflammation, improving cell regeneration, decreasing itching and irritation, and speeding up the skin healing process. In addition, red light therapy is a safe, non-invasive approach, without the common side effects associated with more aggressive treatments.

Red-light therapy has been shown to be beneficial in promoting bone health and preventing osteoporosis, a disease characterized by decreased bone density and impaired bone structure. Red light can stimulate bone formation and strengthen bone density through several mechanisms.

Exposure to red light stimulates bone cells called osteoblasts, which are responsible for the formation of new bone tissue. Red light activates the mitochondria of these cells, which in turn increases cellular energy production (ATP). This increase in energy promotes the synthesis of collagen and other components necessary for the formation of strong and healthy bones.

Red light therapy may also help prevent osteoporosis by inhibiting the activity of osteoclasts, the cells responsible for bone resorption. By regulating the activity of osteoclasts, red light helps maintain an appropriate balance between bone formation and breakdown, resulting in better bone health and less loss of bone density. In addition to preventing osteoporosis, red light therapy can speed the healing process of bone fractures.

Red light stimulates collagen production and promotes cellular regeneration, which can speed fracture healing and reduce recovery time.

The benefits of red light therapy in promoting bone health and preventing osteoporosis include increasing bone density, improving bone strength and structure, and speeding up the healing process of fractures. Importantly, red light therapy should be used as an adjunct to a healthy lifestyle that includes a balanced diet and regular exercise.

DEVICES AND TECHNIQUES

Research has shown that light in the red and near-infrared spectrum (almost red) offers numerous benefits for the body. This light, which typically ranges in frequencies from 620 nanometers (nm) to approximately 1000 nm, has the ability to penetrate deeply into the body's tissues and is highly absorbed by the organism. This range of light, from 600 to 1000 nm, constitutes only a small portion of the electromagnetic spectrum, as illustrated below:

In fact, this portion includes only a minimal fraction of the visible light spectrum that we perceive with the naked eye, along with a small part that is invisible.

Light sources such as the sun and regular incandescent bulbs emit light across all spectrums of visible light, earning them the name "full-spectrum light." This is why a red light therapy device produces a reddish glow, whereas the sun emits white light perceived as yellow. The 660 nanometers appear as a dark red, while the 850 nanometers are invisible.

It is important to note that short-wave infrared light, around 800-1000 nm, is not visible to the naked eye, but it is considered part of the "spectrum" of red light therapy due to its health benefits.

Traditional incandescent bulbs, such as incandescent or halogen bulbs, emit red light, but they also generate a significant amount of heat along with a broad wavelength band. They are less effective for specific therapeutic effects compared to LED lamps. Additionally, these bulbs heat up considerably, limiting the amount of time one can stay close to them.

It is important to note that not only the color of light (wavelength) is crucial but also the amount of light emitted (power density) and the duration of exposure.

Let us delve into detail on what types of red light devices we have available and which ones are most suitable.

TYPES OF RED LIGHT DEVICES

In the field of red light therapy, it is essential to understand the distinct types of devices available. Each device has specific characteristics that can influence its effectiveness and therapeutic applications. Here, the importance of understanding these types of devices is highlighted:

Diversity of devices: There is a wide range of red light devices on the market, including full spectrum lamps, red light panels and portable devices. Understanding the differences between them will allow selecting the most appropriate device for therapeutic and personal needs.

Specificity of treatment: Each type of device may have specific therapeutic applications. By understanding the different devices, doctors can identify which one is most appropriate for the desired treatment. For example, full-spectrum lamps may be beneficial for skin conditions, whereas wearable devices are better suited for localized relief of muscle ailments.

Technical features: Each device has unique technical features such as light wavelength, output power and area coverage. These characteristics may influence the penetration of light into tissues and the effectiveness of treatment. Understanding these technical characteristics is essential to selecting a device that meets specific therapeutic needs and goals.

Devices play a crucial role in red light therapy, as they are the primary tool for managing red light in a controlled and effective manner. Here are some of the reasons why devices are critical in red light therapy:

Accurate management: The devices allow accurate red light management in terms of intensity, duration, and frequency. This is important to ensure that the right amount of red light is provided to obtain the desired therapeutic benefits.

Customization of the treatment: The devices offer the flexibility to customize the treatment according to individual needs. By adjusting device parameters, such as intensity or time of exposure, red light therapy can be tailored to address specific conditions or achieve particular therapeutic goals.

Safety and convenience: The devices are designed with the safety and comfort of the user in mind. For example, they may include eye protection features to prevent possible damage or discomfort during therapy. In addition, wearable devices provide the convenience of using red light therapy at home or on the move, which increases accessibility and adherence to treatment.

Technological advances: Continued innovation in red-light device technology has improved the effectiveness and efficiency of therapy. Technological advances have led to the development of more powerful, compact, and versatile devices, which expands the possibilities of application and improves therapeutic results.

In addition, understanding the distinct types of red light devices also helps avoid potential risks or undesirable outcomes. Each type of device has its own characteristics and limitations, and choosing the wrong device or using it inappropriately can decrease the effectiveness of treatment or even cause unwanted side effects.

For example, if a low-quality device or an inappropriate wavelength is used, red light may not penetrate enough into tissues to provide the desired therapeutic benefits. Similarly, a high-powered device or excessive exposure to red light can cause skin irritation or burns.

In addition, some people may have specific medical conditions or individual sensitivities that require additional precautions when choosing a red light device. For example, those with specific eye disorders, such as diabetic retinopathy or macular degeneration, should be careful when selecting a device and follow medical recommendations to avoid possible damage or worsening of the eye condition.

In general, understanding the diverse types of red light devices helps make informed and safe decisions when choosing the right device for therapy. This involves considering factors such as the condition to be treated, patient comfort, medical recommendations, and technical characteristics of the device. By doing so, you can maximize the effectiveness of treatment and minimize the associated risks.

RDE LIGHT BULBS

Full spectrum red light lamps are devices designed to emit specific wavelength red light, covering the entire spectrum necessary for therapeutic benefit. These lamps use LED or laser technology to generate high intensity and concentrated red light.

In terms of operation, these lamps emit red light at a wavelength generally between 600 and 900 nanometers, which has been shown to penetrate fabrics at different depths. This red light stimulates cellular mitochondria, leading to improved cellular energy production and a number of beneficial biological responses.

Full spectrum red light lamps offer a number of advantages and therapeutic applications. Some of them include:

Improving health and cell regeneration: Full spectrum red light can increase the production of ATP (adenosine triphosphate) in cells, which improves cell function and promotes tissue regeneration and repair.

Relief of pain and inflammation: Red light therapy has been successfully used to relieve pain and reduce inflammation in a variety of conditions, including arthritis, sports injuries, muscle and joint pains, and inflammatory disorders.

Improving skin health: Red light can stimulate the production of collagen and elastin in the skin, which can help reduce wrinkles, improve skin texture, decrease the appearance of scars, and promote a more youthful overall appearance.

Improving athletic performance: Red light therapy can help speed muscle recovery after intense exercise, reduce recovery time, and improve physical performance in athletes and athletes.

When selecting a full-spectrum lamp for home red light therapy, it is important to consider the following considerations:

Light quality and power: Opt for a lamp that offers high quality red light and sufficient power to penetrate tissues properly. It checks the wavelength of the light emitted and the intensity of the lamp output.

Coverage area: Make sure the lamp can cover the desired area for treatment. Some lamps offer a more punctual focus, while others have a wider scattering angle to cover a larger area.

Safety Features: Check if the lamp has safety features, such as overheating protection and automatic shutdown, to prevent injury or damage caused by prolonged or improper use.

Ease of use: Consider the ease of use and lamp configuration options. Some lamps may have predefined settings for different therapeutic applications, while others may be simpler and require manual adjustments.

RED LIGHT PANELS

Red light panels are devices consisting of multiple LED lights or red light lasers that are distributed over a large panel. These panels emit high-intensity red light and can cover larger areas of the body compared to other forms of red light devices.

Red light panels offer a number of benefits in red light therapy. Some of its highlights include:

Wide coverage: Due to their panel-like design, red light panels can cover larger areas of the body, allowing for more extensive exposure to therapeutic light in a single session.

Deep penetration: Red light panels typically have greater power and ability to penetrate into tissues, allowing them to reach deeper layers of skin and muscles for more effective therapeutic results.

Reduced treatment time: Due to their wide coverage area and increased power, red light panels can reduce the time needed to complete a therapy session, which is convenient and efficient for users.

Red light panels are used in a wide range of therapeutic applications. Some common uses include:

Muscle recovery and reduction of inflammation: Red light has been shown to be effective in accelerating muscle recovery after intense exercise and reducing tissue inflammation.

Skin Health Improvement: Red light panels are used in cosmetic treatments to improve skin health and appearance, reducing wrinkles, scars, spots, and other signs of aging.

Pain relief: Red light therapy has been used to relieve pain in various conditions, including arthritis, sports injuries, chronic pain, and musculoskeletal disorders.

Improved sports performance: Red light panels are used in athlete recovery and preparation to improve physical performance, reduce fatigue, and accelerate muscle recovery.

When choosing a red light panel, it is important to consider the following factors:

Power and wavelength: Verifies the output power and wavelength of the light emitted by the panel. The potency should be sufficient to achieve the desired therapeutic effects, and the wavelength should be compatible with existing clinical investigations and studies.

Size and settings: Evaluate the size of the panel and its settings to make sure it fits the areas you want to address. Some panels may have a more flexible or adjustable configuration to suit various parts of the body.

Construction quality and durability: Verify that the panel is made of durable and quality materials to ensure its longevity and optimal performance over time

PORTABLE DEVICES

Portable red light devices are compact and lightweight devices that emit therapeutic red light in the form of LED lights or lasers. These devices are designed to be used conveniently in different areas of the body and are easy to transport and store.

Most portable red light devices consist of a control unit containing LED lights or lasers, as well as a battery or power source. Some devices may have a hand-held design, whereas others may have a headband, panel, or even face mask shape.

Portable red-light devices offer several advantages in red-light therapy:

> Portability: The main advantage of these devices is their portability. You can take them with you to various places and use them in specific areas of the body that require red light therapy.

> Convenient use: Portable devices are easy to use and do not require complicated configuration. You can apply the red light directly to the desired area without the need for bulky cables or equipment.

> Localized application: These devices allow you to precisely target and direct red light on specific areas of the body that need therapy, such as joints, muscles, or skin areas.

Common uses of portable red-light devices include:

> Pain relief: You can use these devices to relieve pain in specific areas of the body, such as painful joints or tight muscles.

Muscle recovery: Portable red light devices are used in muscle recovery after intense exercise, speeding recovery and reducing muscle pain.

Skin treatments: These devices are also used in skin treatments, such as reducing wrinkles, scars, or acne.

When selecting a portable red light device, consider the following considerations:

Power and wavelength: Verifies the output power and wavelength of the light emitted by the device. Make sure that the power is sufficient to achieve the desired therapeutic results and that the wavelength is compatible with existing research and clinical studies.

Size and design: Evaluate the size and design of the device. Make sure it is compact and ergonomic enough for comfortable use and easy handling in the areas to be treated.

Power source: Consider the device's power source, whether it is a rechargeable battery or batteries. Check battery life and easy recharging or replacement of batteries.

By considering these considerations when choosing a portable red light device, you can find one that fits your needs and gives you an effective and safe experience in red light therapy.

CLINICAL BOOTHS

Red light booths are larger devices designed to provide wider exposure to the body and are used in clinical settings such as medical offices, spas, or therapy centers. These arrays are typically equipped with multiple full-spectrum lights or high-intensity LED lights that emit therapeutic red light.

The operation of the red light booths is similar to that of other red light devices, but their design allows for more extensive coverage of the body. Patients are placed inside the cabin, exposing most of their skin to red light for a set period of time.

Red light booths are used for a variety of therapeutic applications, such as:

Treatment of dermatological conditions: Red light can help improve skin health by reducing inflammation, stimulating collagen production, and promoting wound healing. It has been used to treat conditions such as acne, psoriasis, scars, and wrinkles.

Mood therapy and sleep disorders: Exposure to red light can have positive effects on mood by increasing serotonin production and regulating circadian rhythms. It has been used in the treatment of mood disorders such as seasonal depression and in the regulation of sleep.

Muscle recovery and pain relief: Red light can help reduce inflammation, increase blood flow, and speed muscle recovery after intense exercise. It has also been used to relieve pain in specific areas of the body, such as the joints or muscles.

When using red light booths in clinical settings, it is important to consider the following considerations:

Professional supervision: It is recommended that therapy in red light booths be performed under the supervision of a trained health professional, such as a doctor or therapist. They can provide a proper and personalized evaluation, as well as adjust therapy parameters according to individual needs.

Exposure time and frequency: The duration and frequency of exposure to red light in the clinic cabins should be determined by a health care professional. Therapy may vary depending on the condition to be treated and the individual patient's response.

Eye and body protection: Due to the intensity of the light emitted in the cabins, it is important to wear suitable eye protection glasses to prevent eye damage. In addition, extra precautions may be taken to protect sensitive areas of the body, such as the genitals.

Contraindications and precautions: As with other red light devices, it is important to consider the contraindications and precautions specific to each patient before using the red light booths. Some medical conditions, such as light sensitivity or certain eye disorders, may require additional precautions or even contraindicate the use of cabin therapy.

It is essential that the red light booths are properly calibrated and maintained to ensure the correct and consistent emission of the therapeutic light. This may include regular review of light sources and replacement of lamps as recommended by the manufacturer.

Because red light cabins are shared among multiple users, maintaining high standards of hygiene and cleanliness is essential. Be sure to follow established protocols for cabin cleaning and accessories used to minimize the risk of infection or cross-contamination.

It is advisable to maintain an adequate record of patients using the red light booths, including information on the duration of exposure, the frequency of sessions and the results obtained. This makes it easier to monitor the patient's progress and helps adjust therapy as needed.

Professional phototherapy teams

Professional phototherapy teams in clinical settings are more advanced and specialized devices designed to deliver high intensity and precision red light therapy. These kits are usually used by health care practitioners in doctors' offices, hospitals, and specialized clinics.

Key features of professional phototherapy equipment include:

Adjustable intensity: These devices allow the intensity of red light emitted to be controlled and adjusted, making it easier to customize treatment according to the patient's specific needs.

Specific light spectrum: Professional equipment typically has a specific red light spectrum that has been shown to be most effective for certain conditions or therapeutic applications.

Ergonomic design: Professional equipment is designed with patient comfort and safety in mind. They can have features such as adjustable brackets, intuitive control panels and cooling systems to prevent overheating.

Professional phototherapy equipment is used in various fields of medicine and therapy for a wide range of applications. Some common medical and therapeutic uses include:

Dermatology: These kits are used to treat skin conditions such as vitiligo, psoriasis, acne, scars and burns. Red light can help reduce inflammation, promote wound healing, and stimulate collagen production in the skin.

Sports medicine: Professional phototherapy teams are used in sports injury recovery, as red light can help speed muscle recovery, reduce pain and inflammation, and improve athletic performance.

Pain therapy: These devices can be used to relieve chronic pain in different areas of the body, such as joints, muscles, and soft tissues. Red light helps stimulate blood circulation and reduce inflammation, which can relieve discomfort and improve patients' quality of life.

Consider the cost of the equipment and make sure it fits your budget. It compares different options in the market and evaluates whether the value offered by the equipment is in line with its price.

Evaluates whether the equipment is versatile and can be used for a wide range of therapeutic applications. Some devices may have additional configuration options and accessories that allow treatment to be tailored to the specific needs of each patient.

Considerations when choosing a red light therapy device

In addition to the above considerations, it is also important to consider other aspects when choosing a device:

Durability and construction quality: Make sure it is made of durable, high-quality materials that ensure long-term performance. Review other users' reviews and opinions to assess the device's durability and reliability.

Size and portability: Consider size and portability. If you plan to use it in different areas of your home or take it with you on your travels, it is important that it is compact and lightweight enough to make it easy to transport and store.

Configuration and adjustment options: Some full-spectrum devices offer specific intensity adjustment options or treatment modes. These options can allow you to customize therapy according to your individual needs or preferences.

Certifications and approvals: Check for safety certifications and relevant regulatory approvals. This can give you peace of mind regarding the quality and safety of the device.

Warranty and Customer Service: Investigate warranty policies and customer service provided by the manufacturer. Strong warranty and good customer service can be indicative of the manufacturer's confidence in your product and commitment to customer satisfaction.

SECURITY FIRST

POSSIBLE SIDE EFFECTS

Although red light therapy is generally considered safe, it is important to consider possible side effects and contraindications to ensure safe and effective treatment.

First, it is important to recognize that the side effects of red light therapy are usually minimal and temporary. Some people may experience light sensitivity, eye irritation, or minor skin discomfort during or after therapy sessions. These side effects usually disappear quickly and do not pose a significant health risk.

However, absolute, and relative contraindications must be considered before starting red light therapy. Absolute contraindications are situations where red light therapy should under no circumstances be performed. Examples of absolute contraindications may include specific eye disorders, active skin infections, or pregnancy without physician approval. In these cases, it is important to look for safe and appropriate therapeutic alternatives.

On the other hand, relative contraindications are conditions or circumstances in which additional precautions must be taken or a medical evaluation is required before initiating red light therapy. Examples of relative contraindications include clotting disorders, use of photosensitive drugs, or a history of skin cancer. In these situations, it is essential to consult a trained physician or therapist to accurately assess the adequacy of red light therapy and provide personalized recommendations.

Here are some of the possible side effects and situations where red light therapy may not be appropriate:

> a) Sensitivity to light: Some people may experience sensitivity to light, which may manifest as eye irritation or headache. In such cases, it is recommended to wear eye protection during red light therapy.

> (b) Burns and skin lesions: If red light therapy is incorrectly administered or a low-quality device is used, there is a risk of burns or skin lesions. It is important to follow the manufacturer's instructions and make sure that the device meets the appropriate safety standards.

> c) Eye disorders: Direct exposure of the eyes to bright red light can be harmful, especially for people with certain eye disorders, such as cataracts or macular degeneration. In such cases, additional precautions should be taken, including the use of appropriate eye protectors during therapy.

> d) Photosensitive medicines: Some medicines can make the skin more sensitive to light. If you are taking any photosensitive medicines, it is important to consult your doctor before starting red light therapy to evaluate possible contraindications.

There are certain situations where red light therapy is contraindicated and should not be performed under any circumstances. These absolute contraindications indicate that red light therapy may be harmful or not recommended in certain cases. The following are examples of absolute contraindications:

Specific eye disorders: Red light therapy is contraindicated in people who have certain eye disorders, such as advanced glaucoma or severe diabetic retinopathy. These conditions can make the eyes especially sensitive to bright light and may increase the risk of eye damage.

Active skin infections: If there is an active skin infection, such as a bacterial, viral, or fungal infection, red light therapy is contraindicated. Exposure of infected skin to red light may worsen the infection or spread it to other areas of the body.

Pregnancy without doctor approval: During pregnancy, it is essential to get a doctor's approval before performing any type of therapy, including red light therapy. Although no known adverse effects have been reported in connection with red light therapy during pregnancy, caution is required due to the lack of comprehensive studies in this area.

It is important to note that this list of absolute contraindications is not exhaustive and may vary according to the individual medical situation.

There are conditions and circumstances in which additional precautions should be taken or a medical evaluation is required before initiating red light therapy. These are known as relative contraindications, meaning that while red light therapy may be used, special care and medical supervision should be taken. Below are some examples of relative contraindications:

Coagulation disorders: If you have clotting disorders, such as hemophilia or are taking anticoagulant medicines, caution should be exercised when performing red light therapy. Bright light can increase blood flow in the skin and nearby tissues, which may pose an additional risk of bleeding or bleeding. It is important to consult a doctor to assess your individual situation and determine whether red light therapy is safe for you.

Use of photosensitive medicines: Some medicines can make the skin more sensitive to light. These photosensitive medicines may include certain antibiotics, antidepressants, diuretics, and medicines to treat skin conditions. If you are taking any photosensitive medicines, it is important to inform your doctor or therapist before starting red light therapy. Adjustments in the dose or timing of medicinal products may be necessary to avoid potential adverse reactions.

Skin cancer history: If you have a history of skin cancer, especially in the area to be treated, caution should be exercised when performing red light therapy. Stimulating the skin in bright light may have unknown or unwanted effects on cancer cells. In such cases, a thorough medical evaluation is recommended to determine the safety and appropriateness of red light therapy.

Hereditary photosensitivity: Some people may have increased sensitivity to light overall because of hereditary conditions such as protoporphyric erythropoiesis or xeroderma pigmentosum. These conditions can make the skin extremely sensitive to light, which could increase the risk of side effects during red light therapy. Consultation with a specialist physician is essential to determine whether red light therapy is safe in such cases and whether additional precautions are required.

Please note that the above list of relative contraindications is not exhaustive and may vary depending on the individual medical situation. If you have any underlying medical concerns or conditions, it is always advisable to seek the advice of a healthcare professional before starting red light therapy. This will ensure that the necessary precautions are taken and the treatment is customized to maximize the benefits and minimize the potential risks.

SAFE USE

To ensure the safe use of red light therapy devices, certain guidelines and precautions should be followed. Here are some important tips:

a) Read and follow the instructions: It is essential to carefully read the manufacturer's instructions before using any red light therapy device. Follow the recommendations on session length, application distance, and specific advice for your condition or therapeutic purpose.

b) Check the quality of the device: Make sure that the device you are using meets safety and quality standards. Check if you have certifications and endorsement from recognized bodies.

c) Avoid overexposure: Do not exceed the duration or frequency of red light therapy sessions. Follow the manufacturer's recommended guidelines or your therapist's instructions to avoid any risk of overexposure.

d) Avoid sensitive areas: Avoid applying red light directly on sensitive or damaged areas of the skin, such as open wounds, burns or skin rashes.

Tips for effective and safe red light therapy

In addition to the above precautions, here are some general tips to ensure effective and safe red light therapy:

a) Consult a health professional: It is always advisable to consult a health professional, such as a doctor or a therapist, before starting any red light therapy. They will be able to assess your individual medical situation and provide you with appropriate recommendations.

b) Maintain hygiene: Make sure the skin is clean and dry before applying red light therapy. This helps to optimize the absorption of light and reduces the risk of infections or irritations.

c) Be consistent: To obtain optimal results, it is important to be consistent in applying red light therapy. Follow the treatment plan recommended by your therapist and be consistent in the frequency and duration of sessions.

d) Monitor results: Track changes and improvements in your condition as you progress in red light therapy. If you experience any unusual side effects or do not notice improvement after a reasonable time, consult your health care professional.

It is essential to remember that each individual is unique and may have different medical needs and circumstances. Therefore, it is always advisable to seek the advice of a health professional before initiating any type of red light therapy and follow guidelines specific to your particular situation.

INTEGRATION OF RED LIGHT THERAPY IN THERAPEUTICAL PRACTICE

RED LIHT THERAPY AS COMPLEMENTARY

Red light therapy has the potential to integrate with other complementary therapies, which can generate therapeutic synergies and improve outcomes for patients. This integration can encompass a wide range of therapeutic approaches and contribute to a more comprehensive and holistic approach to health care. Here are some ways in which red light therapy can be integrated with other complementary therapies:

(a) Physical therapy and rehabilitation: Red light therapy can complement physical therapy and rehabilitation programs by accelerating recovery from muscle and joint injuries. Red light can help reduce inflammation, relieve pain, and promote tissue regeneration. Combining red light therapy with therapeutic exercises and rehabilitation techniques can improve treatment effectiveness and speed recovery.

b) Acupuncture: The combination of red light therapy and acupuncture may be beneficial. Red light can be applied to acupuncture points during an acupuncture session, enhancing the therapeutic effects of both modalities. Red light can stimulate blood circulation, relieve muscle tension, and improve nervous system response, complementing the balancing and regulating effects of acupuncture.

c) Massage Therapy: Red light therapy can be combined with therapeutic massage to improve the benefits of treatment. Red light can penetrate into tissues and stimulate blood circulation, relax muscles, and reduce tension. By using red light therapy together with proper massage techniques, synergistic benefits can be obtained, accelerating muscle recovery, relieving pain, and promoting relaxation.

(d) Ozone therapy: Ozone therapy, which involves the administration of medicinal ozone, can also be combined with red light therapy. Ozone has anti-inflammatory, antioxidant and regenerative properties and can enhance the therapeutic effects of red light. This combination may be especially beneficial in the treatment of chronic conditions, muscle injuries and degenerative diseases.

e) Relaxation and wellness therapies: Red light therapy can be integrated into relaxation and wellness therapies, such as meditation, aromatherapy, or sound therapy. Red light can provide a relaxing atmosphere and promote a sense of calm and well-being. Combination with these therapies may increase benefits in terms of relaxation, stress reduction, and mood improvement.

It is well known that the integration of red light therapy with complementary therapies should be based on the assessment and experience of the health professional. Each case and patient are unique, so a personalized approach adapted to individual needs is required. Collaboration among different health professionals can be essential to achieve an effective and safe integration of these complementary therapies.

THE FUTURE OF RED LIGHT THERAPY

TECHNOLOGICAL PROGRESS AND TRENDS

In recent years, red light therapy has undergone significant advances that have expanded its applications and improved its effectiveness. Here are some of the most recent and relevant developments in this field:

Increased wavelength accuracy: Researchers have been able to further fine-tune red light emission in terms of its specific wavelength. This has allowed for greater precision in stimulating biological processes and a better understanding of the underlying mechanisms. In addition to conventional red light, the use of other wavelengths within the near-red spectrum, such as near-infrared light, has also been explored and has shown promising effects on therapy.

Development of wearable devices: Previously, red light therapy was carried out mainly in clinics or medical offices, using large and expensive devices. However, technological advances have allowed the development of portable and more accessible devices for home use. These devices are smaller, more comfortable to use, and offer the possibility of home therapy, which has increased the convenience and availability of treatment for patients.

Intelligent control and monitoring systems: Intelligent control and monitoring systems have been introduced in red light therapy devices. These systems allow light intensity and duration to be precisely adjusted, as well as real-time monitoring of patient responses. By combining advanced algorithms and sensor technologies, these intelligent systems can tailor therapy to individual patients' needs, thereby improving treatment effectiveness and outcomes.

Integration with other complementary therapies: There has been a growing interest in combining red light therapy with other complementary therapies, such as physical therapy, acupuncture, and massage therapy. This integration seeks to enhance therapeutic effects and provide a more holistic approach to the treatment of various conditions. Combined therapies can expand treatment options and offer synergistic benefits for patients.

Aesthetic and regenerative medicine applications: Red light therapy has found promising applications in the field of aesthetic and regenerative medicine. It has been used to improve the appearance of the skin, reduce wrinkles, and fine lines, and promote wound healing and cell regeneration. Clinical studies have supported the benefits of red light therapy in skin rejuvenation and stimulation of hair growth, leading to its adoption in aesthetic clinics and spas.

These recent advances in red light therapy demonstrate immense potential for improving people's health and well-being.

FUTURE PROSPECTS FOR RESEARCH AND DEVELOPMENT

Red light therapy has captured the attention of researchers and designers, leading to the exploration of innovative applications and cutting-edge designs. These new ideas seek to maximize the effectiveness of therapy and offer more convenient and personalized solutions for patients. Here are some of the potential innovative applications and designs that could define the future of red light therapy:

(a) Portable clothing devices: Advances in smart textiles are expected to enable the integration of red light therapy into clothing. For example, shirts or jackets with optical fibers that emit red light could be developed, allowing continuous, discreet exposure to therapy during the day. These wearable devices may be especially useful for managing chronic conditions or for improving general well-being.

(b) Red light therapy in mobile devices: As smartphones and tablets have become ubiquitous, it is expected that red light therapy will be integrated into mobile applications and accessories. Users could use their device to receive personalized red light treatments, with the ability to adjust the intensity and duration according to their needs. This would increase accessibility and allow people to conduct therapy anytime, anywhere.

(c) Virtual reality red light therapy: Combining red light therapy with virtual reality could offer an immersive and therapeutic experience. Using virtual reality glasses equipped with integrated red lights, patients could receive treatments while immersing themselves in relaxing or stimulating virtual environments. This combination of red light and virtual reality therapy could improve efficacy by leveraging the synergistic effects of both modalities.

(d) Red light therapy on sports grounds: Professional and amateur athletes are constantly looking for new ways to improve their performance and accelerate recovery. In this sense, it is expected that red light therapy will be integrated into sports grounds, gyms, and training centers. Teams and athletes could use high-powered red lights to stimulate muscle recovery, improve endurance and reduce injury time.

(e) Red light therapy in the field of neurology: As the understanding of how red light affects the brain deepens, innovative applications in the field of neurology are being explored. Preliminary research has suggested that red light therapy may have positive effects on neurodegenerative diseases such as Alzheimer's and Parkinson's. In the future, specific devices for red-light brain stimulation may be developed, which could have a significant impact on the treatment of these conditions.

Technological advances and emerging trends in red light therapy have the potential to offer a number of significant benefits for patients and healthcare professionals. These advances can improve the effectiveness of therapy, increase accessibility, and provide more personalized options. Customization and adaptability are key elements in red light therapy, and technological advances are enabling greater flexibility and precision in the design of personalized treatments. As the effects of red light on the human body are better understood, therapy parameters can be adjusted to suit the individual needs of each patient.

As red light therapy becomes more popular, it is important to establish regulations and quality standards to ensure the safety and efficacy of devices and treatments. This implies the need for adequate oversight by regulatory bodies and the implementation of responsible manufacturing and marketing practices.

CONCLUSIONS AND FINAL TIPS

In this book, we have thoroughly explored the various aspects of red light therapy and its application in the field of health and wellness. We have understood that red light, with a specific wavelength, has the ability to penetrate skin layers and reach underlying tissues and cells, triggering beneficial biochemical and therapeutic responses.

We have examined the biological effects of red light therapy, such as stimulating cell energy production, improving blood circulation, tissue regeneration, and influencing the production of hormones and neurotransmitters. In addition, we have explored its application in different areas of health, such as the management of mood disorders, sleep disorders, pain, skin care, among others.

For therapists interested in red light therapy, it is critical to consider the following recommendations:

Understand the science: Become familiar with the basic principles of red light therapy, including mechanisms of action, appropriate doses, and recommended treatment protocols.

Stay updated: Stay on top of research and advances in the field of red light therapy to deliver the best results to customers.

Customize treatments: Each individual may respond differently to red light therapy, so it is important to tailor treatments to the specific needs and conditions of each patient.

Working collaboratively: Consider red light therapy as a complementary tool in the context of a holistic approach to health and wellness. Working in partnership with other health care practitioners to provide a holistic, multidisciplinary approach

Maintain safety: Ensure that safety guidelines recommended by manufacturers of red-light devices are followed and provide appropriate guidance on eye protection and other necessary precautions.

Red light therapy has proven to be a promising therapeutic modality in various areas of health and well-being. As we continue to research and better understand the underlying mechanisms, their applications are expanding.

When researching and using red light therapy, obtaining informed consent from patients, and ensuring that ethical principles are followed in the research are essential. This involves providing clear and understandable information about the risks and benefits of therapy, as well as respecting the autonomy and privacy of clinical trial participants.

It is important to recognize that red light therapy is not a substitute for conventional medical care, but a complementary tool that can offer additional benefits.

Also, it is essential that therapists be committed to scientific evidence, safety, and ethics in their practice.

Although promising research supports the benefits of red light therapy, it is important to continue advancing scientific research to fully understand its effectiveness in different medical conditions. Well-designed clinical studies and robust data are crucial to support therapeutic claims and ensure patient safety.

RESEARCH AND EVIDENCE

Barolet, D. (2008). Light-emitting diodes (LEDs) in dermatology. Seminars in Cutaneous Medicine and Surgery, 27(4), p. 227-238.

Avci, P., Gupta, A., Sadasivam, M., Vecchio, D., Pam, Z., Pam, N., & Hamblin, M. R. (2013). Low-level laser (light) therapy (LLLT) in skin: Stimulating, healing, restoring. Seminars in Cutaneous Medicine and Surgery, 32(1), 41-52.

Wunsch, A., & Matuschka, K. (2014). A controlled trial to determine the efficacy of red and near-infrared light treatment in patient satisfaction, reduction of fine lines, wrinkles, skin roughness, and intradermal collagen density increase. Photomedicine and Laser Surgery, 32(2), 93-100.

Desmet, K. D., Paz, D. A., Corry, J. J., Eells, J. T., & Wong-Riley, M. T. (2006). Mitochondrial gene expression in response to light therapy. Photomedicine and Laser Surgery, 24(2), p. 229-235.

Naeser, M. A., Zafonte, R., Kengel, M. H., Martin, P. I., Frazier, J., Hamblin, M. R., ... & Hamblin, M. R. (2014). Significant improvements in post-transcranial, red/near-infrared light-emitting diode treatments in chronic, mild traumatic brain injury: open-protocol study. Journal of Neurotrauma, 31(11), 1008-1017.

Ferraresi, C., Hamblin, M. R., & Parizotto, N. A. (2012). Low-level laser (light) therapy (LLLT) on muscle tissue: performance, fatigue and repair benefited by the power of light. Photonics & Lasers in Medicine, 1(4), 267-286.

Schiffer, F., Johnston, A. L., Ravichandran, C., Polcari, A., Teicher, M. H., Webb, R. H., ... & Hamblin, M. R. (2009). Psychological benefits 2 and 4 weeks after a single treatment with near-infrared light to the forehead: a pilot study of 10 patients with major depression and anxiety Behavioral and Brain Functions, 5(1), 46.

"The Effects of Red Light on the Mitochondria" - This article, published in the journal Nature in 2018, analyzes the molecular and cellular mechanisms of how red light affects mitochondria and its involvement in health and aging.

"Photobiomodulation in human muscle tissue: an advantage in sports performance?" - Published in the journal Sports Medicine in 2018, this article reviews the scientific evidence on the effects of red light therapy on athletic performance and muscle recovery.

"The Use of Low-Level Light Therapy in Dermatology: A Critical Review" - Published in the journal Dermatologic Surgery in 2017, this article examines the use of red light therapy in skin care and its effectiveness in the treatment of various dermatological conditions.

"Low-level laser (light) therapy (LLLT) on muscle tissue: performance, fatigue, and repair benefited by the power of light" - This article, published in Photonics & Lasers in Medicine in 2012, highlights the benefits of red light therapy on muscle performance, fatigue, and recovery.

"The potential of light therapy in Parkinson's disease" - Published in the journal Neuroscience and Biobehavioral Reviews in 2016, this article examines the use of red light therapy in the treatment of Parkinson's disease and its potential to improve motor and non-motor symptoms.

ABOUT SUSAN MCDOWELL

In the dynamic world of health and wellness, Dr. Susan McDowell stands out as a visionary and a beacon of knowledge, profoundly dedicated to empowering individuals to reach their full potential. Her journey in medicine is not merely a career, but a lifelong pursuit of understanding and sharing the intricacies of human well-being.

Dr. McDowell's foundational expertise was forged at the prestigious University of Medicine and Health Sciences, where she earned her medical degree. This rigorous academic background laid the groundwork for a professional path characterized by a unique blend of hands-on clinical expertise and an unwavering commitment to research. For years, she has cultivated her own medical practice, earning not only the respect but also the deep admiration of her patients through her compassionate care.

Beyond the clinic, Susan McDowell has forged an innovative path as a prolific writer, extending her influence far beyond individual consultations. Her extensive writings are a testament to her profound medical knowledge, yet they offer something more: they distill her innate compassion and unwavering dedication to continuously improving the health and well-being of all who seek her guidance. Her publications resonate deeply, reflecting an integrative approach that has made meaningful contributions to the field. While the sources don't specify all her topics, the mention of "Going barefoot" alongside her medical background hints at the breadth and diverse nature of her explorations within health and wellness, reflecting her prolific output.

Through both her clinical practice and her impactful written works, Susan McDowell has firmly established herself as a highly respected figure in the expansive field of health and medicine, a testament to her holistic vision and relentless dedication. She truly embodies the spirit of a leading medical professional, constantly pushing the boundaries of knowledge for the betterment of others.

Beyond her impressive credentials and extensive knowledge, Dr. Susan McDowell's approach to healthcare is deeply rooted in her profound empathy and a genuinely warm, welcoming demeanor. Her clinical practice is more than just a place for medical consultation; it is a space where her deep passion for helping people reach their full potential truly shines through. This innate drive translates into an environment where patients feel not just treated, but genuinely understood and cared for.

Dr. McDowell's personal philosophy distills her compassion and unwavering commitment to the continuous improvement of the health and well-being of those who seek her guidance. It is this patient-centered approach, marked by a welcoming spirit and an admirable dedication, that has earned her not just the respect, but the deep admiration of her patients over many years in her own practice. While the sources primarily highlight her interactions with patients and those who seek her guidance, her demonstrated compassion and dedication suggest an intrinsically warm and supportive professional persona.

OTHER BOOKS BY THE AUTHOR

"Andropause Exposed: The Hidden Male Menopause, Low Testosterone, and the Secret to Reclaiming Energy, Strength, and Confidence"

The groundbreaking book, "Andropause Exposed: The Hidden Male Menopause, Low Testosterone, and the Secret to Reclaiming Energy, Strength, and Confidence," offers a comprehensive, empathetic, and empowering guide to understanding, managing, and thriving through these changes.

"Parenting without fear: A Guide to Loving Your Children"

Are you tired of parenting approaches rooted in anxiety, control, or endless struggles? For generations, many parenting practices have been influenced by underlying fears: fear of children not learning, not behaving, or not succeeding. These methods, often relying on pressures, rewards, or anger, can be not only ineffective but also deeply detrimental to a child's intrinsic drive for self-development. In 'Parenting without Fear,' we invite you to embark on a revolutionary journey that challenges conventional wisdom and reconsiders the very foundation of how you guide your children.

"Going barefoot: natural running, walking and movement to respect your body"

In "Going Barefoot: Natural Running, Walking and Movement to Respect Your Body," Susan McDowell delves into the profound benefits of reconnecting with the earth through natural movement. This insightful book emphasizes the importance of barefoot activities in fostering alignment, strength, and overall well-being. Drawing from both scientific research and her rich clinical experience, Susan offers practical advice and exercises to help readers embrace a more natural way of moving.

"Understanding SIBO: The Enigma of Small Intestinal Bacterial Overgrowth".

This book, the result of Susan's clinical experience, offers a clear and practical perspective on Small Intestinal Bacterial Overgrowth Syndrome (SIBO). Through her work, Susan unravels the mysteries of this condition, providing readers with an essential guide to understanding, addressing, and overcoming SIBO.

"Understanding Perimenopause: A Woman in Plenitude"

Discover the beauty in every change, from hormonal aspects to symptoms and body changes. With personal stories and anecdotes that resonate, you will feel accompanied in this unique chapter of your life. It explores how sexual health, emotional and psychological aspects, and general well-being intertwine in a journey full of authenticity and self-acceptance.

"Complete Guide to Red Light Therapy: Optimal Health, Healthy Skin and Other Benefits of Red Light."

As an advocate of holistic approaches to health, Susan explores the diverse benefits of red-light therapy in this book. From improving skin health to optimizing overall wellness, Susan's comprehensive guide offers valuable information backed by research, allowing readers to effectively integrate red light into their daily routine.

"Microdosing: Macrobenefits in health and well-being. Your body in psychedelic and non-psychedelic substances."

In her most innovative work, Susan explores the fascinating world of microdosing and its impacts on health and wellness. This book provides a balanced and scientifically grounded view on the use of psychedelic and non-psychedelic substances in microdosing, offering a unique perspective on their potential benefit to mental and emotional health.

"High-Need Babies, The Untold Truth: The Ultimate Parenting Guide for High-Demanding Childs (English Edition)"

Susan McDowell embarks on the journey of parenting with her English-language play "High-Need Babies." This book provides a unique and comprehensive insight for parents facing the challenge of raising children with high demands. With empathy and wisdom, Susan guides parents through effective strategies and offers an enlightening perspective on the particular needs of these children.

MAGAtations:

Guided Meditations for a Stronger, United America

Written by Ald
Published by Dizzy-Angel Multimedia

CONTENTS

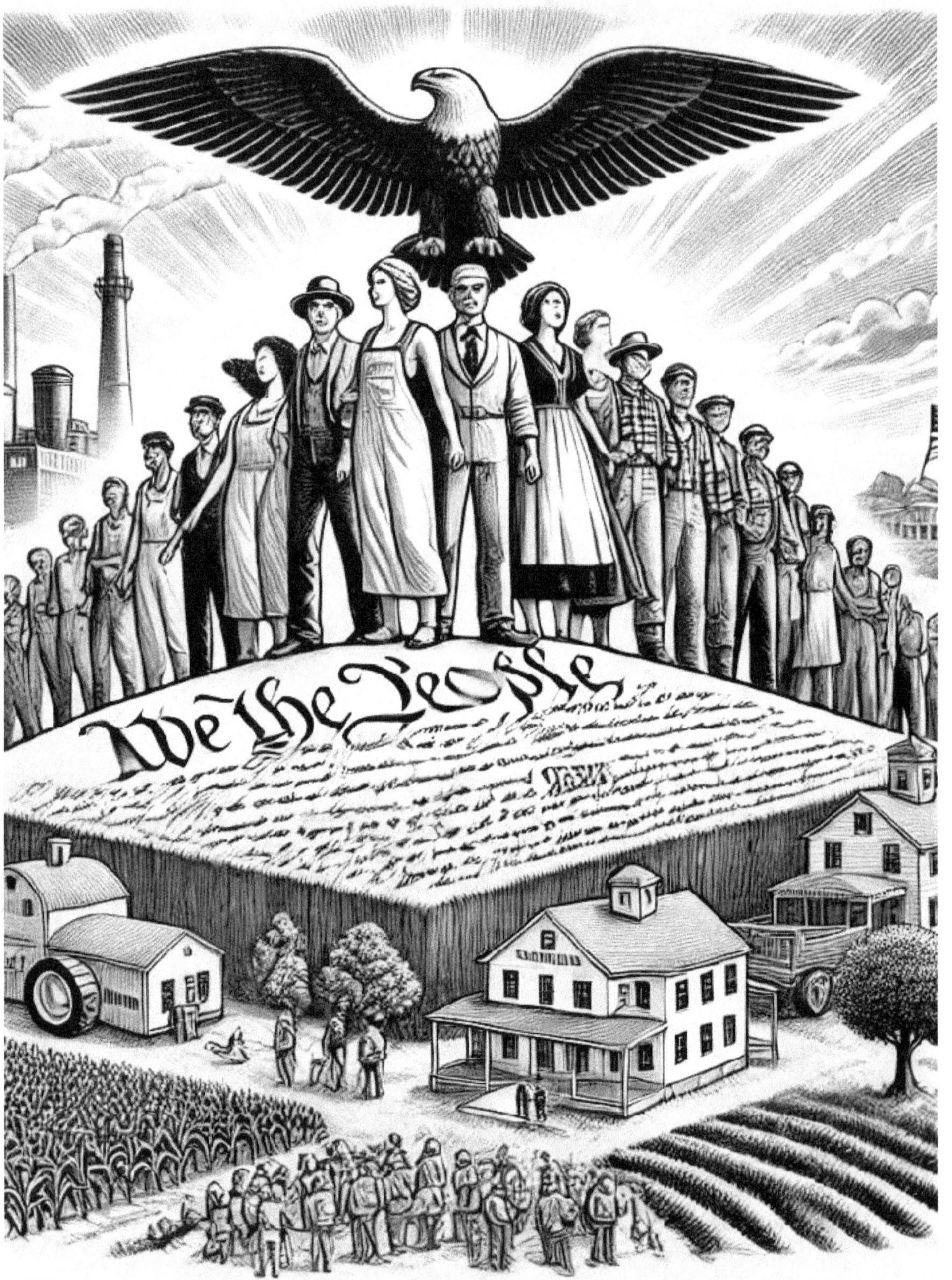
We The People

Introduction

America has always been a land of ideals—a country built on the promise of freedom, the pursuit of opportunity, and the power of individuals to shape their destinies. Yet, these ideals often feel tested as times change and challenges arise. For millions of Americans, the MAGA movement represents a rallying cry to preserve and strengthen the principles that make the nation exceptional. This book is a tribute to that vision, an invitation to reflect on these priorities, and a guide for meaningful action to support a brighter future.

The MAGA movement is more than a political perspective; it is a deeply held set of values that resonates with people from all walks of life. It emphasizes the importance of American workers and industries, the sanctity of Constitutional rights, the need for secure borders, and the preservation of national sovereignty. These beliefs are rooted in recognizing that a strong, united America benefits its citizens and the world. The movement is driven by a profound respect for the individual, a love of freedom, and a commitment to protecting the institutions and traditions that uphold them.

This book seeks to honor these priorities while providing a compassionate and thoughtful space for reflection. Each section delves into one of the core issues that define the movement, from economic growth and energy independence to election integrity and healthcare reform. These topics are presented with balance and inclusivity, offering insights into how these values can unite people in a common purpose rather than divide them.

Each section is accompanied by guided meditations, affirmations, journaling prompts, and actionable steps designed to inspire personal reflection and practical engagement. This format encourages readers to deepen their understanding of these issues and feel empowered to contribute to the changes they wish to see. Whether you seek clarity, strength, or direction, these tools help guide your journey.

Central to this book is the belief that positive change begins with individuals and families. Economic strength, secure communities, and thriving families are not abstract goals but profoundly personal and interconnected. A family that finds security through stable work, a community that benefits from local energy production, or a nation that upholds the rule of law contributes to everyone's collective well-being. These values are the foundation of a society that believes in the dignity of every person and the potential of every community.

We also recognize the challenges inherent in today's complex world. Concerns about government overreach, healthcare affordability, or election transparency reflect a desire for fair, accountable, and trustworthy systems. These challenges are not insurmountable; they are opportunities for innovation, collaboration, and moral solutions. This book encourages readers to approach these issues not with anger or fear but with hope, clarity, and determination.

This is not a book about division. It is a book about unity through shared values—celebrating the resilience, innovation, and compassion that define the American spirit. It is a call to action to build bridges between individuals and communities, protect the freedoms we cherish, and embrace the future with optimism and resolve.

As you read, reflect, and engage with the content of this book, may you feel inspired to strengthen the values you hold dear and share them in ways that bring people together? May this book be a companion in your pursuit of understanding, purpose, and meaningful change.

Together, we can strengthen the bonds that unite us, celebrate the principles that define us, and work toward a future where every American has the opportunity to thrive. The journey begins with respect, reflection, and action and starts here.

What This Book IS

This book is a guide, a resource, and a source of inspiration for those who care deeply about the values that shape our nation and their lives. It is thoughtfully crafted to offer clarity, focus, and empowerment, helping readers engage with essential issues meaningfully and productively. Here's what this book *is*:

This book addresses topics that matter to millions of Americans—economic growth, constitutional rights, election integrity, energy independence, and more. These discussions are presented respectfully, focusing on shared values and constructive approaches to complex challenges. Each section delves into the heart of the issue, offering insights and context that encourage understanding and thoughtful engagement.

In a world full of distractions, roadblocks, and diversions, it can be challenging to concentrate on the issues that truly matter. This book includes guided meditations that help readers quiet the noise and focus on what's essential. These meditations are designed to inspire clarity and resilience, providing a grounding force amid the chaos of political and cultural discourse.

Each section includes affirmations to uplift and empower the reader. These affirmations serve as reminders of the strength and potential within each individual, reinforcing the belief that positive change begins with personal growth and focused action. By affirming their values and goals, readers are encouraged to approach challenges with confidence and hope.

The book includes journaling prompts in every section to help readers deepen their understanding of the issues and connect with their values. These prompts encourage thoughtful exploration, allowing readers to "flesh out" concepts, ideas, and emotions. Through reflection, readers can identify how these issues impact their lives and how they might take meaningful action to address them.

Each section concludes with an inspiring wrap-up that ties together the ideas presented and offers actionable steps for readers. These conclusions are designed to motivate readers and equip them to make a difference in their personal lives, communities, or the nation.

This book celebrates focus, resilience, and the power of shared values. It guides staying true to the principles that matter most, free from the distractions and divisive rhetoric that can cloud judgment. By combining thoughtful discussion with tools for personal growth and empowerment, this book offers a pathway to clarity and purpose—a way forward that honors both the individual and the greater good.

What This Book Is NOT

In today's highly charged political climate, it's easy to assume that any discussion of key national issues must take sides, provoke controversy, or stir division. This book is intentionally designed to do none of those things. Instead, it seeks a respectful, thoughtful, and uplifting exploration of values that matter to millions of Americans. To set clear expectations, here is what this book is *not*:

While the issues discussed in this book resonate with many who identify with the MAGA movement, this is not a rallying cry for populist ideology. It is a reflective guide intended to promote personal growth, constructive action, and community empowerment—offering practical tools to approach shared concerns with thoughtfulness and balance.

This book is written with respect for diverse perspectives and avoids partisan rhetoric. It does not seek to critique, demean, or vilify those with different political views. Instead, it focuses on the values and goals that unite Americans and provides space for reflection and understanding, regardless of political affiliation.

Controversy often dominates public discourse, but this book seeks a different path. It fosters connection and hope, focusing on shared values like economic opportunity, individual freedom, and community well-being. This book is about what brings us together, not what tears us apart.

This book addresses the integrity of elections through the lens of trust, transparency, and fairness without delving into specific allegations or controversies. The goal is to inspire confidence in the democratic process and encourage constructive engagement, not to stoke division or revisit past grievances.

Instead, this book guides those who care deeply about family, faith, freedom, and the nation's future. It offers practical, actionable ways to reflect on and address our challenges while fostering unity, respect, and hope. It is a celebration of values and a call to action for a brighter tomorrow—free from the noise and conflict that too often dominate the conversation.

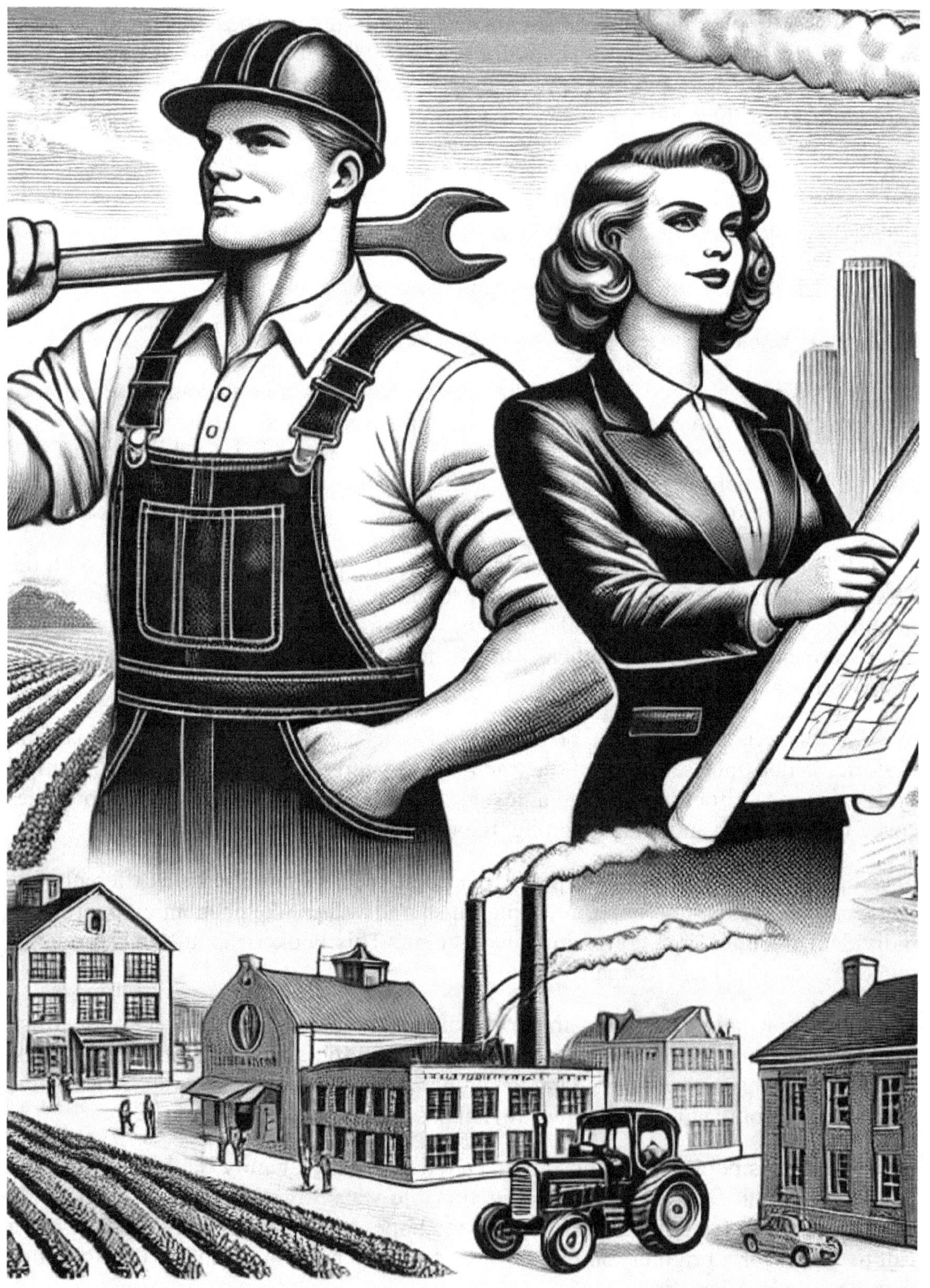

ONE: Economic Growth and Job Creation

America has long been celebrated as a land of opportunity, where hard work and ingenuity pave the way for prosperity. However, recent years have seen growing concerns about economic challenges, from job outsourcing to stagnant wages and the decline of once-thriving industries. Addressing these concerns means prioritizing policies championing American workers, revitalizing manufacturing, and returning jobs to the United States. This section explores how these efforts strengthen the economy and restore community hope, pride, and resilience.

Manufacturing has always been a cornerstone of the American economy, providing stable jobs and fostering innovation. However, globalization has led to significant outsourcing of production, leaving behind empty factories and struggling communities. Revitalizing domestic manufacturing means investing in infrastructure, reducing business barriers, and ensuring that "Made in the USA" symbolizes excellence. By supporting policies that encourage local production, we create jobs that sustain families and communities while strengthening national self-reliance.

Innovation and entrepreneurship are powerful drivers of economic growth. American ingenuity fuels progress and creates opportunities, from small businesses to cutting-edge startups. Encouraging these ventures means providing access to capital, reducing unnecessary regulations, and fostering a culture that celebrates risk-taking and creativity. When individuals are empowered to pursue their ideas, they generate jobs, inspire others, and contribute to a thriving economy.

At the heart of economic growth are the workers who make it possible. Supporting American workers involves advocating for fair wages, equitable working conditions, and access to training programs that prepare them for the evolving demands of the job market. As industries adapt to new technologies and global trends, investing in education and workforce development ensures that workers remain competitive and equipped to succeed. By championing policies prioritizing workers, we honor their contributions and secure a prosperous future for all.

Economic growth isn't just about numbers on a national scale—it's about revitalizing local communities. When factories reopen, small businesses flourish, and families find meaningful work, the benefits ripple. Strong local economies contribute to better schools, safer neighborhoods, and tighter-knit communities. Prioritizing policies that empower states and regions to harness their unique strengths helps rebuild the fabric of struggling areas, ensuring that no part of the country is left behind.

Economic growth and environmental stewardship can coexist. As we revitalize industries and create jobs, adopting sustainable practices that protect the environment for future generations is essential. Investing in cleaner technologies and renewable energy drives innovation and ensures that growth is balanced with responsibility. By prioritizing sustainability alongside economic progress, we demonstrate that prosperity and preservation go hand in hand.

Embracing American Resilience

Why It Matters:

America's enduring strength shines brightest during times of hardship. Generation after generation, workers across this nation have encountered daunting challenges—economic downturns, global competition, and evolving industries—yet have emerged with renewed purpose. This resilience isn't just about survival; it's about adapting, innovating, and forging new paths that ensure our economy stays dynamic, inclusive, and sustainable. By embracing this spirit of perseverance, we help guarantee that America remains a place where hard work is rewarded, communities prosper, and opportunity abounds.

From the family-owned machine shop in a small Midwestern town to the bustling factory floors of America's industrial heartland, hardworking men and women carry a legacy of ingenuity and grit. By prioritizing policies that invest in domestic manufacturing, skill development, and fair competition, we reinvigorate our production capabilities and restore confidence to American workers. Recognizing and fostering our resilience ensures that we don't merely return to the past—we forge a future defined by strength, self-reliance, and a commitment to passing these values on to future generations.

Guided Meditation:

Find a quiet, comfortable place where you can fully relax. Close your eyes and take three deep breaths, inhaling possibility and exhaling doubt. Imagine yourself stepping into a bright, humming workshop—its floors clean, its tools organized, and its workers moving with focused determination.

Observe the smooth rhythm of machinery as skilled hands transform raw materials into finely crafted products. Each spark of light from a welding torch speaks of human ingenuity; each carefully measured cut is a sign of steady hands shaped by years of practice. Envision the workers' faces: some young, others lined with experience, all united by a quiet pride that says, "We can do this."

With each breath, you absorb this energy of resilience and adaptability. You feel the strong current of tradition and perseverance flowing through you, connecting you to generations of Americans who never gave up. It's as if their willpower is your own, guiding you to stand taller and face challenges head-on.

As you continue to breathe steadily, imagine shelves lined with goods proudly labeled "Made in the USA," each item a testament to the skill and devotion behind it. Feel gratitude for these people, this place, and your role in continuing this legacy. When you're ready, gently open your eyes, reassuring you that American resilience lives in you, fueling your aspirations and strengthening your resolve.

Affirmation:

"I am part of a legacy of resilience and carry the spirit of American perseverance and adaptability."

Journaling Prompts:

Think of a time when you faced a setback or challenge in your work or personal life. How did you adapt, and what did you learn from the experience?

Write about a person or group you admire for their perseverance and innovation. How can their story inspire your approach to challenges?

Envision your community to thrive economically with new jobs and opportunities. What steps could you, as an individual, take to help bring about that vision?

Practices in Action:

Support Local Businesses: Make a conscious effort to purchase goods produced by local craftspeople and U.S. manufacturers. Investing in their success helps sustain jobs and strengthens your community's economic fabric.

Skill Building: Whether you're learning a trade, honing a craft, or mentoring someone starting, commit to personal or community skill development. These investments ensure a steady pipeline of talented workers ready to face economic challenges head-on.

Conclusion:

By embracing American resilience, we honor those who came before us and lay the groundwork for a more secure and prosperous tomorrow. Recognizing our capacity to adapt, innovate, and thrive under pressure allows us to build an economy supporting hardworking families and uplifting communities. It embodies the timeless virtues that have guided America through every challenge it has ever encountered.

Rekindling Domestic Manufacturing:

Why It Matters:

Reviving America's domestic manufacturing isn't just about bringing back jobs; it's about restoring a sense of purpose, quality, and craftsmanship to our everyday lives. When we support products "Made in the USA," we strengthen the ties between workers, communities, and the marketplace, building an economy that values durability and American know-how. This isn't about turning back the clock to a bygone era—it's about blending time-honored skills with modern innovation to ensure a stable future for American industries.

Local factories, workshops, and artisan studios help communities thrive. Each well-paying manufacturing job spurs local growth, encourages entrepreneurship, and creates a ripple effect that benefits schools, healthcare systems, and small businesses. By renewing our commitment to producing goods at home, we affirm that value isn't measured solely by profit margins; it's also found in the pride workers take in their craft and the satisfaction customers feel knowing their purchase supports their fellow Americans. Embracing domestic manufacturing means embracing the American worker's skill and dedication, forging a path toward greater independence and prosperity.

Guided Meditation:

Find a quiet place to relax, close your eyes, and take three slow, calming breaths. Imagine yourself stepping onto a warm, well-lit factory floor. Machines hum steadily, and the scent of freshly cut wood or forged steel fills the air.

Notice a group of workers skillfully assembling a product. Their hands move confidently and purposefully, each part fitting precisely into place. Listen to the gentle chorus of tools as they craft something sturdy, something meant to last. This is not disposable work—this is a labor of dignity.

As you breathe in, feel the pride and satisfaction flowing from these workers into you. See their careful craftsmanship reflected in their faces, each proud to be part of something meaningful. With every breath, you absorb that pride and the understanding that domestic manufacturing isn't just an industry—it's a way of affirming the American spirit.

Before opening your eyes, imagine shelves filled with these locally made goods, since the care that went into each item and its positive impact on local communities. Carry this respect and admiration with you as you return to the present, knowing that reviving domestic manufacturing nurtures economic stability and national pride.

Affirmation

"I honor the skill of American craftsmanship, and by supporting domestic manufacturing, I help strengthen our communities and nation."

Journaling Prompts:

Reflect on a product you own that was made in the USA. What qualities make it stand out, and how does it feel knowing it supports American workers?

Consider the skills and trades that once thrived in your local area. How might they be revived, and what would that renewal mean for your community?

Envision a future where Americans increasingly value quality and craftsmanship. How can you contribute to making that vision a reality?

Practices in Action:

Buy Local, Buy American: Whenever possible, choose products made in the USA. Over time, these small decisions can create greater demand for domestic goods, fueling local growth.

Celebrate Craftsmanship by Attending local fairs, visiting artisan workshops, or contacting neighbors who run small manufacturing businesses. Showing support and learning about their work inspires others to appreciate and invest in homegrown talent.

Conclusion:

By rekindling domestic manufacturing, we restore dignity and stability to American workplaces. We reaffirm that our workforce's quality, ingenuity, and skill can be the backbone of a thriving economy. In standing up for local industries, we celebrate the idea that a robust future lies not in outsourcing our strength but in nurturing it right here at home—one handcrafted product at a time.

Honoring the American Worker's Legacy

Why It Matters:

America's economic story is woven from the threads of countless workers who have shaped our nation's prosperity. The hardworking Americans who built our railroads, constructed our skyscrapers, farmed our lands, and assembled our machines forged a legacy of determination and skill. By connecting current job creation efforts to this enduring heritage, we acknowledge that every modern achievement stands on the shoulders of generations who dared to dream, build, and improve our nation's economic landscape.

We better understand the value of investing in our future when we recognize how far we've come. Today's policies and initiatives aim to cultivate a workforce that honors the past by carrying its torch forward. Just as previous generations overcame challenges to innovate, we too can embrace new opportunities to ensure that Americans continue to thrive in every industry, from traditional manufacturing to cutting-edge technology. This mindful appreciation of our past serves not as nostalgia but as inspiration—fueling a workforce ready to meet the moment and prepare a brighter future for all.

Guided Meditation:

Find a quiet, comfortable position and close your eyes. Take three deep, centering breaths. Imagine standing in front of a timeline that stretches far into the past. Each moment in American economic history—each pioneering invention, each flourishing industry—glimmers with meaning and effort.

Gently step forward along this timeline. Hear the echoes of hammers striking steel, the hum of assembly lines, the laughter and chatter of breakrooms and family dinners after long shifts. Feel the warmth and wisdom of those who came before—immigrants, innovators, parents, and mentors who worked tirelessly to provide for their families and secure a better life.

As you continue along the timeline, notice how these past achievements flow naturally into the present. Our modern workplaces, bustling job sites, and creative startups are not isolated—they're the latest chapter in a living story. With each breath, absorb the understanding that your contributions add new pages to this legacy.

Now, slowly return to the present moment. Carry with you the knowledge that your efforts matter. You continue a heritage of perseverance and adaptability. As you open your eyes, feel gratitude for those who came before and a sense of responsibility to honor their sacrifices through your dedication and initiative.

Affirmation:

"I honor the work and sacrifice of past generations, and by building upon their legacy, I strengthen America's future."

Journaling Prompts:

Reflect on a family member or historical figure whose hard work helped shape your opportunities today. How does their story inspire you?

Consider what values and lessons you'd like to pass on from past generations. What elements of their legacy can guide your own career and life choices?

Imagine looking back to the future. What contributions do you hope will become part of the American worker's legacy because of your actions today?

Practices in Action:

Learn Your Community's Economic Story: Visit local museums, read about regional industries, or talk with elders who can share their experiences. Understanding local history fosters a deeper connection to your community's future.

Mentor or Volunteer: Offer guidance to young people starting their careers or those learning new trades. Passing along knowledge and inspiration keeps our legacy of hard work, skill, and determination alive.

Conclusion:

By honoring the American worker's legacy, we recognize that our opportunities and successes are not ours alone—they're part of a continuous narrative. Acknowledging past sacrifices and achievements, we find fresh determination to uphold timeless values. In respecting where we came from, we gain clarity about where we're going, building an America that future generations will be proud to inherit.

Cultivating Local Prosperity:

Why It Matters:

Local prosperity isn't just about economics—it's about ensuring communities maintain their character, values, and purpose. Small towns, rural communities, and once-bustling industrial areas regain their unique identities when local economies thrive. Instead of watching talent drift away to distant cities or overseas opportunities, these regions nurture the next generation of builders, entrepreneurs, and innovators right at home.

By investing in strong local economies, we encourage more than just financial stability. We foster environments where families feel secure, main streets regain their vibrancy, and neighbors support one another through shared commitment and pride. Cultivating local prosperity ensures that American communities remain lively and self-sufficient, ready to adapt to new challenges and opportunities.

Guided Meditation:

Find a quiet space, sit comfortably, and close your eyes. Take three slow, steady breaths, inhaling strength and exhaling stress. Imagine yourself standing at the center of a small town's main street. The morning sun warms the pavement, and a gentle breeze carries the scent of fresh coffee from a nearby café.

Look around and see local shops and businesses: a family-owned hardware store, a bakery whose recipes span generations, and a small manufacturing plant that provides steady jobs. Notice how people greet one another by name, smiling and exchanging stories. There is a shared confidence here—an understanding that everyone's success feeds into the community's greater good.

As you breathe in, feel the pride and stability that come from meaningful, local work. These are not distant industries run by invisible boards; these are neighbors, friends, and families dedicated to uplifting each other. With every breath, absorb the assurance that communities become resilient, adaptable, and independent when they create their paths to prosperity.

Before opening your eyes, imagine the next generation stepping confidently into this scene—young adults finding careers close to home, children dreaming of their future businesses, elders passing down knowledge and tradition. Carry this vision forward: a future where towns, large and small, define their destinies and thrive on the strength of their people.

Affirmation:

"I support the growth of local communities, knowing that strong hometown economies create stability, pride, and opportunity for all."

Journaling Prompts:

Reflect on a local business or industry from your hometown. What impact has it had on your community's spirit and well-being?

Consider the changes you want to see in your local economy. What types of jobs, services, or opportunities would help it flourish?

Imagine being part of a community-wide effort to revitalize your area's prosperity. How would you contribute, and what positive changes would you hope to inspire?

Practices in Action:

Shop Local First: Support nearby businesses and industries before looking elsewhere. Your choices help keep money circulating within the community, strengthening local jobs and services.

Engage in Community Building: Attend town hall meetings, volunteer at local events, or join economic development groups. Your involvement conveys that the community's future matters and that everyone has a role.

Conclusion:

Cultivating local prosperity affirms that opportunity doesn't always come from distant places—it can be nurtured right where we stand. By supporting hometown businesses, encouraging young entrepreneurs, and contributing to community life, we help revitalize small towns, rural communities, and industrial hubs alike. In doing so, we ensure that the heart of America continues to beat strong, vibrant, and full of promise.

Nurturing Entrepreneurship & Innovation:

Why It Matters:

The entrepreneurial spirit has long been the lifeblood of America's economic vitality. It's not limited to towering corporations or Silicon Valley tech giants—innovation springs from small workshops, family-owned farms, and local garages, where an idea and a bit of determination can spark something extraordinary. Embracing entrepreneurship means encouraging risk-takers, dreamers, and problem-solvers at every level of society, ensuring our economy evolves, adapts, and expands.

By nurturing new ideas and supporting local startups, we foster a climate where anyone with courage and ingenuity can turn their vision into reality. This approach empowers communities, stimulates healthy competition, and makes our economy more resilient. It acknowledges that the best solutions often emerge when creative minds have the freedom, support, and resources to flourish.

Guided Meditation:

Sit comfortably and close your eyes. Take three deep, steady breaths, inhaling innovation and exhaling limitation. Imagine stepping into a brightly lit studio or workshop, where tools and materials line the walls, and ideas seem to shimmer in the air.

Look around and see individuals of all ages and backgrounds brainstorming, testing prototypes, and perfecting their craft. Each person brings unique experiences and talents, transforming challenges into opportunities, hesitation into confidence, and raw potential into tangible creations.

As you inhale, feel the spark of their creativity flow into you. Imagine their enthusiasm, willingness to try something new, and resilience in the face of setbacks. With every breath, you absorb the certainty that you, too, can contribute to the grand tapestry of American innovation.

Before you open your eyes, envision the fruits of these labors spreading across the nation—local economies strengthened, new jobs created, and solutions to problems once thought insurmountable. When you return to the present, carry with you the assurance that American ingenuity thrives in the hearts of everyday people, ready to uplift communities and inspire growth.

Affirmation:

"I honor the creative spark that fuels American innovation, and I trust my ability to contribute to a future defined by entrepreneurial spirit and resilience."

Journaling Prompts:

Reflect on when you or someone you know risked to start something new. What lessons emerged from that experience?

Consider one area in your community that could benefit from fresh ideas or improved services. How might you or others spark the innovation needed to meet that need?

Write about your untapped ideas or passions. What small steps could you take today to nurture your entrepreneurial spirit?

Practices in Action:

Support Local Entrepreneurs: Visit local craft fairs, try out new small businesses, or invest in local startups through community programs. Your support helps promising ventures gain footing.

Mentor and Network: If you have professional experience, consider offering guidance to a budding entrepreneur. If you want to start something yourself, contact local business associations or innovation hubs that can provide advice and resources.

Conclusion:

Nurturing entrepreneurship and innovation ensures that America remains where dreams don't merely linger—they take shape and grow. We foster an economy that rewards creativity, hard work, and courage by supporting local inventors and visionaries. The result is a more dynamic and inclusive marketplace where every new idea promises a better, stronger, and more prosperous nation.

Fostering Community Through Employment:

Why It Matters:

Stable, meaningful employment isn't just about a steady paycheck—it's about nurturing the social fabric that holds communities together. When people have reliable jobs close to home, families experience more stability, and neighborhoods benefit from increased engagement and cooperation. This economic security strengthens our social bonds, creating an environment where children can grow up knowing the value of hard work, neighbors look out for one another, and local traditions thrive.

By linking job creation to stronger families and connected communities, we recognize that economic policies have far-reaching implications. It's not only about wages and productivity; it's also about building places where people care, contribute, and invest their time and energy. In fostering community through employment, we ensure that economic growth uplifts everyone, leaving no family or neighborhood behind.

Guided Meditation:

Find a comfortable space, close your eyes, and take three deep, calming breaths. Envision yourself strolling through a familiar neighborhood. Notice the sound of children playing, the hum of conversation on front porches, and the warm glow of lights in family-owned shops. There's a sense of comfort and security in the air.

Walk down the street and see people returning home from work—some wearing uniforms, others carrying briefcases or toolkits. Each of them contributes not just to their livelihood but to the prosperity of the entire community. Their stability weaves a strong social net, holding families close and allowing friendships to flourish.

As you breathe steadily, feel yourself absorbing the harmony from knowing everyone's effort matters. The well-being of one strengthens the whole, and each job planted here, in this shared hometown soil, grows into a more vibrant, nurturing environment.

Before opening your eyes, picture the generations thriving there. Envision children growing into confident adults, supported by the opportunities and goodwill seeded today. With a final deep breath, carry the understanding that meaningful work binds neighbors, families, and friends into a resilient, united community.

Affirmation:

"I recognize that every stable job strengthens the bond between families, neighbors, and friends, helping our communities grow closer and more resilient."

Journaling Prompts:

Reflect on how meaningful work has influenced your family or neighborhood. How have stable jobs helped foster trust, cooperation, and a shared purpose where you live?

Consider someone in your life who found new confidence or improved well-being through meaningful employment. How did their personal growth ripple out to those around them?

Envision a future in which every family in your community has access to secure, fulfilling work. What would your neighborhood feel like, and how might relationships deepen and flourish?

Practices in Action:

Support Local Hiring Efforts: Patronize businesses that prioritize local workers and consider how your hiring decisions (if applicable) can uplift people in your area.

Volunteer & Connect: Get involved in community programs that help people find employment, develop job skills, or improve their resumes. Your contribution could be the key to someone's gain of stability and confidence.

Conclusion:

Fostering community through employment acknowledges that economics and social well-being are intertwined. By championing job creation that respects human dignity and strengthens neighborhoods, we build a society where everyone has a place to belong and flourish. Investing in secure, meaningful work doesn't just lift individuals—we ensure that the entire community grows more potent, closer, and hopeful for the future.

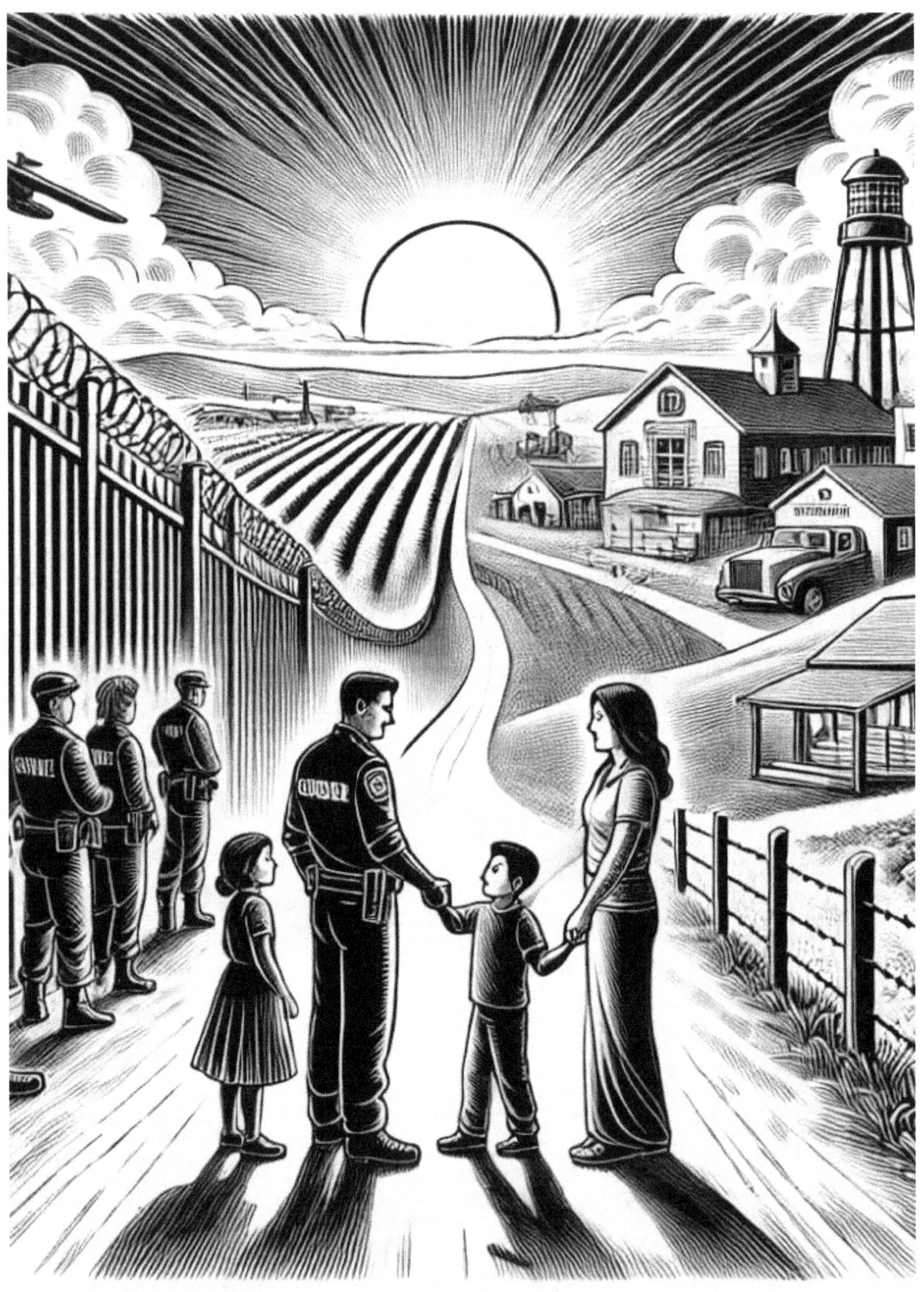

TWO: Border Security and Immigration

A secure border is essential to preserving a nation's sovereignty and safety. For centuries, America has been a beacon of hope and opportunity, welcoming individuals worldwide who seek a better life. Yet, managing this openness requires a balance between compassion and clarity. Immigration policies must respect the rule of law while addressing citizens' needs and concerns. A strong focus on border security safeguards not only the integrity of the immigration system but also the stability of American communities.

Border security encompasses more than physical barriers—it encompasses advanced technology, well-trained personnel, and coordinated efforts to prevent illegal activity. A secure border protects communities from threats like human trafficking, drug smuggling, and other forms of criminal activity while ensuring that immigration is conducted through lawful and transparent processes. By strengthening border security, we promote stability and uphold the principle that the law applies equally to all.

America's immigration system is most effective when fair, orderly, and consistent. Protecting its integrity means enforcing existing laws, addressing vulnerabilities, and ensuring that those seeking to enter the country do so through legal pathways. Clear and consistent policies support newcomers and long-time citizens by fostering trust, reducing exploitation, and maintaining equality and justice.

While security is essential, so is compassion. America's legacy as a land of opportunity must be honored by creating pathways for legal immigration that reflect both humanitarian values and the nation's economic and social needs. This balance ensures that America remains where individuals can aspire to a better future while respecting the structures that make such opportunities possible. Compassion and clarity are not opposing forces—they are complementary principles that guide effective immigration policy.

A well-functioning border and immigration system strengthens communities, preserves cultural heritage, and ensures fairness for all. When laws are respected, local economies thrive, families feel secure, and neighborhoods grow stronger. Policies prioritizing order and fairness create a foundation for shared success, helping communities embrace diversity while remaining safe and cohesive.

Reaffirming National Sovereignty:

Why It Matters:

A nation's sovereignty is built on the understanding that it governs itself and protects its citizens by setting clear rules and boundaries. Clearly defined borders aren't meant to hinder legitimate movement; they ensure a country can maintain its identity, culture, and institutions. By recognizing the importance of these boundaries, we affirm that every citizen has a stake in how their nation grows, adapts, and engages with the world.

When we reaffirm the principle of national sovereignty, we acknowledge that our shared values, legal frameworks, and responsibilities hold us together. Securing borders assures that the nation's choices—about who enters, who stays, and how resources are allocated—reflect the people's collective will. In a world of shifting alliances and rapid change, upholding sovereignty ensures that America remains true to itself, standing firm on a foundation of mutual respect, trust, and defined responsibility.

Guided Meditation:

Find a quiet, comfortable spot and close your eyes. Take three slow, steady breaths, inhaling confidence and exhaling uncertainty. Imagine looking out across a peaceful landscape—a place you call home, where open fields meet distant hills beneath a clear sky.

As you observe this landscape, envision a gentle but unmistakable boundary that separates your homeland from the wide world beyond. This boundary isn't a barrier to understanding or cooperation; it is a marker that defines who you are, guiding how you welcome others and maintain your way of life.

With each breath, feel a sense of reassurance: just as a family's home has walls and doors to protect those inside, so do a nation's borders to ensure its integrity. Sense the pride, responsibility, and dignity that come from cherishing your homeland's sovereignty.

Before you open your eyes, imagine that this defined border doesn't isolate you from the world—it gives you a place to stand and understand who you are and what you can offer. Carry with you the knowledge that by respecting and securing these boundaries, you nurture your nation's character, unity, and future.

Affirmation:

"I honor the clear boundaries that safeguard our national identity and ensure that we govern ourselves with integrity and purpose."

Journaling Prompts:

Reflect on what national sovereignty means to you. How does having clearly defined borders contribute to a sense of belonging, safety, and cultural continuity?

Consider how a balanced approach to sovereignty can encourage respectful engagement with other nations. How might clear borders foster both cooperation and healthy independence?

Consider what values, traditions, or principles you believe are worth protecting within your nation. How does sovereignty help preserve these ideals for future generations?

Practices in Action:

Stay Informed & Involved: Learn about your nation's immigration policies, border security measures, and diplomatic efforts. Understanding can help shape thoughtful discussions with friends, neighbors, and community groups.

Encourage Civil Dialogue: Engage in respectful conversations about national sovereignty, listening to different perspectives. Support efforts to educate others about the importance of well-defined borders and the rule of law, promoting a balanced and constructive approach.

Conclusion:

Reaffirming national sovereignty ensures that a nation remains true to its principles, upholds its responsibilities, and maintains the integrity of its social and cultural fabric. By establishing and respecting boundaries, we grant ourselves the freedom to shape the future in a way that honors our heritage, welcomes respectful engagement with other nations, and preserves the essence of what it means to be home.

Securing Communities & Families:

Why It Matters:

At the heart of every thriving community is a sense of safety, stability, and belonging. When our borders are enforced responsibly, we create conditions that help preserve the integrity of our neighborhoods. Strong border policies don't just exist in theory—they affect the real lives of families looking to raise children in peaceful surroundings, business owners seeking stable marketplaces, and communities hoping to maintain a positive quality of life.

By establishing and maintaining secure borders, we help ensure that those who enter our country do so through fair, legal, and transparent processes. This structure helps protect against threats such as organized crime and illegal trafficking while reinforcing the rule of law. As a result, American families can enjoy greater security, enabling them to invest in their futures, strengthen their relationships, and nurture communities that genuinely feel like home.

Guided Meditation:

Find a quiet space and close your eyes. Take three slow, calming breaths, inhaling peace and exhaling tension. Imagine standing at the edge of your neighborhood—familiar streets, friendly houses, and a playground where children's laughter drifts on the breeze.

Envision a clear boundary that safely regulates who comes and goes, ensuring your community remains where neighbors look out for one another. This boundary doesn't create fear; it instills trust. Behind it, people greet each other warmly, confident they are protected from hidden dangers that might undermine their shared values.

With each breath, sense the relief from knowing your loved ones can walk these sidewalks safely, that local businesses can flourish without undue threats, and that schools can focus on education rather than managing chaos. Feel the comfort of this structured environment, where the security of the border helps maintain stability within.

Before you open your eyes, imagine children growing up here calmly and optimistically. They inherit a legacy of well-being and mutual responsibility. When you return to the present, carry this awareness with you, knowing that through thoughtful border enforcement, communities and families find the reassurance they need to thrive.

Affirmation:

"I value the security and stability that thoughtful border enforcement brings, preserving the well-being of our communities and families."

Journaling Prompts:

Reflect on the qualities that make your neighborhood feel secure. How might proper border enforcement support those qualities on a national scale?

Consider how a secure environment allows families and communities to focus on growth rather than fear. What does this shift in focus mean for future generations?

Write about a vision of your ideal community. How do fair and consistent border policies contribute to that vision?

Practices in Action:

Stay Informed About Local Impacts: Learn how border policies affect your region through local news, town hall meetings, or community discussions. Understanding the connection between national enforcement and neighborhood safety fosters informed participation.

Support Community Watch & Outreach Programs: Engage in initiatives encouraging neighbors to look out for one another. Strengthening local bonds complements broader security efforts, ensuring everyone plays a part in maintaining a safe environment.

Conclusion:

Securing communities and families through proper border enforcement goes beyond abstract policy debates. It's about crafting an environment where people can confidently lead their lives, invest in their futures, and support one another. We reinforce the foundation for building strong, harmonious neighborhoods by valuing safety and stability.

Upholding Law & Order:

Why It Matters:

A nation founded on principles of law and fairness thrives when it upholds these values in all aspects of life, including its immigration system. By reinforcing rules that are clear, consistent, and applied evenly, we ensure that both longtime citizens and newcomers operate within a framework that respects everyone's rights and responsibilities. A lawful immigration system isn't intended to shut people out—it's meant to establish a fair and transparent process that welcomes those who seek to contribute honestly and honorably.

When we stress the importance of law and order in immigration, we foster trust in our institutions and confidence in our shared future. Communities become places where established residents feel secure in their way of life, and newcomers have the opportunity to integrate smoothly and proudly. Upholding the rule of law empowers everyone—ensuring stability, promoting common standards of conduct, and forging a more unified national identity.

Guided Meditation:

Settle into a quiet, comfortable position and close your eyes. Take three deep breaths, inhaling integrity and exhaling uncertainty. Picture yourself standing at a welcoming entrance to a nation built on shared values. Here, every person knows what is expected and understands the path to belonging.

See newcomers arriving hopeful and determined, carrying their dreams alongside their luggage. Imagine them being greeted by a transparent and orderly process that honors their desire to contribute while upholding the standards that maintain a strong, lawful society.

As you breathe in, feel the steady reassurance from fairness and consistency. Recognize how clarity in rules and regulations affirms the dignity of those seeking entry and preserves the trust of those calling this place home.

Before you open your eyes, envision communities where longstanding residents and new arrivals share meals, traditions, and aspirations. Their mutual respect thrives because everyone has followed an honest, established path. Bring this vision back with you—a reminder that lawful, orderly systems benefit everyone.

Affirmation:

"I support an immigration process built on fairness and accountability, ensuring respect for longtime citizens and newcomers who honor our laws."

Journaling Prompts:

Reflect on when adhering to clear rules benefited everyone involved. How can this principle strengthen our approach to immigration?

Consider the qualities—integrity, respect, patience—that make a lawful immigration system meaningful. How do these values reinforce trust within communities?

Imagine a scenario where newcomers and long-term residents come together as neighbors. How do established processes and shared expectations help foster genuine acceptance?

Practices in Action:

Stay Informed About the Immigration Process: Learn how legal immigration works in the United States, including the steps newcomers must take. This understanding can clarify discussions and help guide constructive conversations.

Promote Fairness & Respect: When discussing immigration in your community, emphasize the importance of abiding by the law while showing compassion. Encourage dialogue that respects the hopes of those seeking a better life and the rights of current citizens.

Conclusion:

Upholding law and order in immigration safeguards our shared values, ensuring trust and respect, and guides how we welcome newcomers. By embracing rules that reward honesty and diligence, we nurture a social fabric where everyone's contributions are valued. Together, we can foster unity, security, and the promise of a brighter tomorrow for all who call this nation home.

Ensuring Economic Fairness:

Why It Matters:

Economic fairness depends on a balance between opportunity and responsibility. When immigration policies are carefully structured to prioritize merit and fairness, they safeguard American workers and ensure that the job market remains stable, competitive, and rewarding. Controlling the flow of new arrivals helps prevent wage suppression and job displacement, supporting a standard of living that benefits both established citizens and future generations.

By creating clear, merit-based pathways for legal immigration, we encourage newcomers who genuinely wish to contribute their skills and dedication to the American economy. This approach rewards effort and integrity, attracting those who add value and respect established rules. In doing so, we uphold a system where citizens and immigrants alike can pursue meaningful, dignified work without the constant fear of unfair competition.

Guided Meditation:

Find a quiet place, close your eyes, and take three calming breaths. Envision an open field where hardworking Americans sow seeds of effort and care, each seeking to reap the fruits of their labor with honesty and perseverance.

Imagine newcomers arriving at the edge of this field, eager to plant their seeds. They do so through a fair, merit-based process—receiving the guidance, tools, and permission to join the cultivation. Each person follows a path defined by mutual respect and established rules, ensuring the harvest remains abundant, not overrun.

As you breathe steadily, feel the harmony that emerges when everyone contributes according to a fair standard. The field remains orderly, productive, and nurturing. Visualize the way this balanced approach to immigration preserves both opportunity and stability.

Before you open your eyes, imagine families, longtime Americans, and newcomers enjoying the harvest together. Their joint efforts create a shared prosperity born of cooperation and fairness. Carry this vision with you, knowing that controlled, merit-based immigration supports economic well-being for all.

Affirmation:

"I believe in an immigration system that safeguards American jobs, rewards diligence, and encourages newcomers who earn their place with integrity."

Journaling Prompts:

Reflect on what a fair job market means to you. How can controlled, merit-based immigration help ensure that everyone has a fair shot at stable employment?

Consider how economic fairness relates to respect for existing citizens and aspiring immigrants. In what ways do clear guidelines uplift everyone involved?

Envision a future in which economic opportunity is widely available and fairly earned. What role does thoughtful, merit-based immigration play in achieving that vision?

Practices in Action:

Support Policy Discussions: Engage in conversations about immigration, focusing on economic fairness and understanding how merit-based reforms can protect jobs and wages. Stay informed on proposed policies and share your insights with neighbors and community leaders.

Encourage Skills Development: Advocate for job training programs and career pathways for citizens and legal immigrants that help everyone compete on a level playing field. Strengthening skills and qualifications contributes to a healthier, more resilient workforce.

Conclusion:

Ensuring economic fairness in immigration policy is about balancing opportunity with responsibility. By setting clear standards and encouraging newcomers to contribute through hard work and merit, we protect American livelihoods and reinforce our national work ethic. In fostering this equilibrium, we secure a brighter, more sustainable economic future built on fairness, dignity, and shared prosperity.

Balancing Compassion with Clarity:

Why It Matters:

Striking the right balance between compassion and clarity at the border acknowledges our shared humanity and the integrity of our national framework. People worldwide seek new opportunities, often driven by desperate circumstances, and America's long tradition has been to welcome those who follow a lawful path. At the same time, we must maintain clear, consistent rules to preserve the stability and security that make this nation a place people want to join.

By pairing compassion with careful enforcement, we ensure that those who legitimately seek a better life can do so with dignity while respecting the laws and principles that protect American communities. This equilibrium honors the individual stories of hope and resilience without compromising the structure that allows our country to remain strong, secure, and guided by shared values.

Guided Meditation:

Close your eyes, settle in, and take three steady breaths. Picture yourself standing at a calm border crossing beneath a soft, early morning light. On one side are families who have followed a process—maybe waiting patiently for years—to begin a new chapter. On the other side stands the nation they hope to join, its rules and expectations posted, ensuring a fair and orderly approach.

Take in the scene of earnest faces, hopeful eyes, and children holding onto their parents' hands. Feel compassion rise within you as you imagine the hardships they might have overcome. Yet, I also sense the quiet strength of the guiding principles that have shaped this country. These rules are not a rejection; they are the framework that makes meaningful, lasting welcome possible.

As you breathe, recognize that compassion and clarity are partners, not opponents. Compassion encourages understanding, patience, and kindness. Clarity ensures everyone follows the same path, preventing chaos and preserving order. Together, they form a stable bridge, allowing those who seek a better life to cross with purpose while safeguarding what makes this nation strong.

Before you open your eyes, envision these families entering through clear, lawful channels. Imagine them embracing new opportunities, contributing their talents, and enriching the tapestry of American life. Carry with you the understanding that genuine compassion flourishes when nurtured within a framework of fairness and consistency.

Affirmation:

"I hold compassion and clarity in harmony, ensuring that goodwill and fair rules guide the journey of those who seek a better life within our nation."

Journaling Prompts:

Recall when you had to balance kindness with maintaining boundaries. How does this experience help you understand the importance of compassion and clarity in immigration?

Consider what values and principles should guide the balance between caring for those in need and enforcing fair rules at the border. How might these values shape future policies?

Envision a scenario where newcomers, welcomed through lawful channels, thrive alongside established citizens. What does this harmonious coexistence look and feel like?

Practices in Action:

Educate Yourself & Others: Learn about legal immigration processes, humanitarian programs, and pathways available to those seeking a new life. Share this knowledge in conversations to foster nuanced, empathetic discussions.

Support Local Organizations: Contribute to community groups or charities that help newcomers navigate the legal processes. Your involvement can embody the spirit of compassion while reinforcing lawful avenues of entry.

Conclusion:

Balancing compassion with clarity at our borders acknowledges that kindness and order are not mutually exclusive. By welcoming people through fair, transparent systems, we preserve our nation's integrity while opening our doors to those who genuinely seek to contribute. This careful blending of care and structure ensures that America remains a beacon of hope rooted in principle, strength, and shared respect.

Honoring the American Tradition of Legal Immigration:

Why It Matters:

America's strength owes much to generations of immigrants who came here with dreams and respect for the nation's laws and ideals. These individuals helped build railroads, open businesses, forge new industries, and enrich our cultural tapestry, all while following established pathways. Honoring this tradition means recognizing that the greatness of our country is rooted in the values and responsibilities embraced by those who arrived and integrated lawfully.

By reaffirming our commitment to legal immigration, we celebrate the newcomers who have contributed their skills and hard work and the long-standing citizens who welcomed them. This legacy of lawful integration reminds us that the United States thrives when individuals seek not to bypass its rules but to uphold them, forging a shared future based on mutual respect, opportunity, and responsibility.

Guided Meditation:

Find a calm, quiet place and close your eyes. Take three steady breaths: Inhale gratitude and exhale distraction. Picture a long timeline stretching before you, each point representing generations of immigrants who traveled far to become part of the American story.

Move along this timeline. See families who arrived decades ago, guided by the lamp of the Statue of Liberty, determined to follow the proper steps to make America their home. Imagine them learning the language, adapting to new customs, and planting seeds of prosperity for themselves and their neighbors.

With each breath, feel a deep appreciation for their willingness to work within our nation's laws. These individuals didn't look for shortcuts but respected the process, ensuring their contributions were rooted in trust and shared commitment.

.As you slowly open your eyes, envision this legacy continuing today. Newcomers still choose to honor America's legal pathways, weaving their hopes and talents into the fabric of our society. Carry forward the understanding that this lawful integration remains a cornerstone of our national character.

Affirmation:

"I respect and celebrate America's legacy of lawful integration, recognizing that we grow stronger when newcomers honor our nation's principles and opportunities."

Journaling Prompts:

Recall a personal or historical story of an immigrant family who followed the legal path to U.S. citizenship. How did their choices shape their future and that of their descendants?

Consider the values of honesty, perseverance, and respect that lawful immigrants uphold. Which of these values resonate most with you, and why?

Envision a future in which legal pathways remain a cherished tradition. How might this reaffirmation strengthen the bond between generations of Americans, both established and new?

Practices in Action:

Learn & Share Stories: Research the journeys of lawful immigrants who helped build your local community. Share their stories with family and friends to inspire greater appreciation for this tradition.

Advocate for Clear Pathways: Support efforts to streamline and clarify legal immigration processes. Encouraging fair, accessible, and transparent steps helps newcomers integrate smoothly, benefiting us all.

Conclusion:

Honoring the American tradition of legal immigration reminds us that our nation's strength is not built on circumventing rules but on living up to them. By cherishing this legacy, we remain faithful to the principles that have guided countless newcomers into productive, enriching lives in the United States. In doing so, we uphold a legacy of lawful integration that continues to enrich our communities, strengthen our economy, and unify us as one people under shared values.

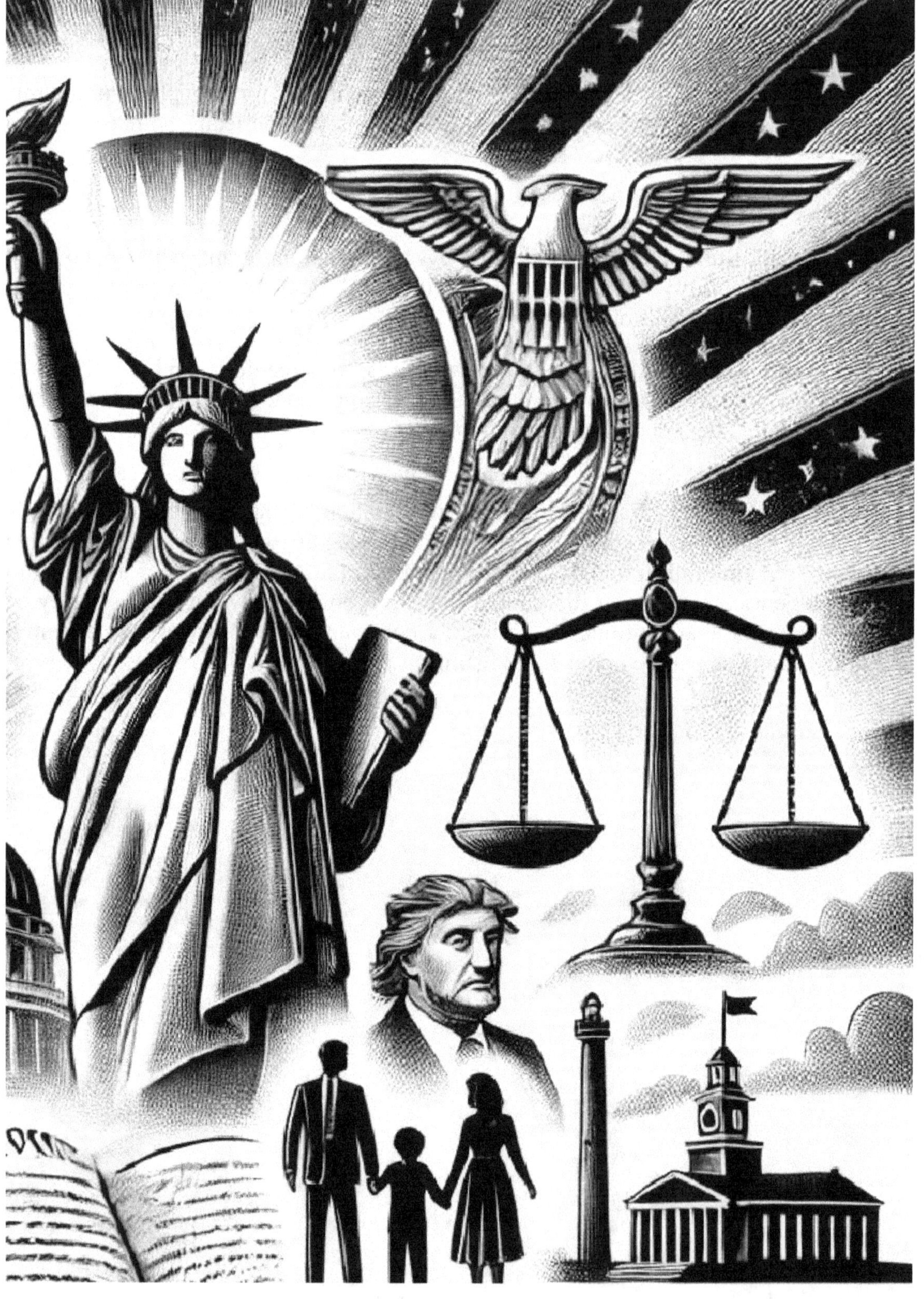

THREE: Preserving Constitutional Rights

The Constitution of the United States is the foundation of American liberty, safeguarding the rights and freedoms that define the nation's character. From the Second Amendment to the protection of free speech and religious freedom, these rights empower individuals, foster diversity of thought, and ensure that every citizen can live with dignity and autonomy. Preserving these rights is not just about honoring the past—it's about securing the principles that make freedom and self-governance possible for future generations.

The Second Amendment is a testament to the enduring spirit of self-reliance and personal security. For many Americans, the right to bear arms symbolizes the freedom to protect oneself, one's family, and property. Preserving this right involves thoughtful advocacy that respects the balance between public safety and individual liberty, ensuring that responsible gun ownership remains a cornerstone of American life.

Free speech is the bedrock of a healthy democracy, allowing individuals to express their ideas, challenge authority, and engage in open dialogue. This freedom fosters innovation, resilience, and progress, even when perspectives differ. Preserving free speech requires vigilance, especially in an era of rapid technological change, to ensure that every voice can be heard without fear of censorship or suppression.

Religious freedom is a profoundly personal right that upholds the ability of individuals to worship—or not worship—according to their own beliefs. This freedom fosters a diverse and pluralistic society where people of all faiths and philosophies coexist respectfully. Protecting religious freedom involves safeguarding this right against interference while promoting understanding and tolerance among all Americans.

The Constitution's system of checks and balances ensures that no single branch of government holds unchecked power. Preserving this structure protects individual rights by holding leaders accountable to the people. Advocacy for Constitutional rights includes defending these mechanisms and ensuring that the principles of fairness and justice remain central to governance.

Preserving Constitutional rights begins with understanding them. Education and civic engagement empower citizens to recognize their rights, advocate for their preservation, and challenge encroachments when they arise. A nation where individuals are informed about their freedoms is better equipped to protect and cherish them.

Honoring the Founding Principles:

Why It Matters:

When the Founding Fathers shaped the United States, they did so with the conviction that individual liberty would form the nation's heart. They carefully crafted a Constitution that safeguarded rights like free speech, religious freedom, and the right to bear arms, ensuring that power would not rest in a distant authority but with the people themselves. Their work wasn't about one moment in time—it was about building a system capable of adapting and thriving as America grew.

By honoring the Founding Principles, we affirm the bedrock of our national character. These principles protect everyday citizens' voices and guarantee that regardless of era, Americans can speak their minds, worship as they choose, and defend themselves and their families. Upholding this legacy isn't a return to the past; it's a way of forging a more substantial future guided by enduring wisdom and respect for the individual spirit.

Guided Meditation:

Find a quiet, comfortable place and close your eyes. Take three deep breaths, inhale gratitude, and exhale distraction. Imagine standing before an old, well-lit hall—its wooden floors gently creak beneath your feet, and portraits of the Founding Fathers on its walls, who debated, deliberated, and designed the framework of American freedoms.

Step into this hall. Hear the soft hum of voices echoing through history. Visualize the Founders—Jefferson, Madison, Franklin—engaged in thoughtful discussion. Their words carry weight and intention. They strived to protect future generations they would never meet, trusting that their ideals would stand the test of time.

With each breath, feel the gravity of what these individuals set into motion: a system where your voice matters, your beliefs can be openly expressed, and your right to defend yourself is enshrined in law. These freedoms aren't abstractions; they are living guarantees, sculpted to endure through changing landscapes and shifting political currents.

Before opening your eyes, imagine a clear light shining upon you and the Constitution itself. Absorb that light, letting it fill you with respect, responsibility, and the understanding that you are a steward of these principles. As you return to the present moment, carry the knowledge that by honoring the Founding Fathers' foresight, you help preserve the cornerstone of American life.

Affirmation:

"I honor the Founders' wisdom and embrace the liberties they secured, preserving the enduring ideals that shape our American experience."

Journaling Prompts:

Reflect on a constitutional right you value deeply. How does this right shape your daily life, decisions, or sense of security?

Consider the debates and compromises the Founders made. How might understanding their intentions help guide us when facing modern challenges?

Imagine explaining America's founding principles to someone unfamiliar with our history. Which core values would you emphasize, and why?

Practices in Action:

Learn & Share: Read one of the founding documents—the Constitution, the Bill of Rights, or the Federalist Papers—and discuss your insights with friends or family. Spreading understanding helps keep these principles alive.

Engage in Civic Life: Attend local meetings, vote in elections, or join community groups that protect constitutional rights. Your participation ensures these liberties remain more than words on parchment.

Conclusion:

By honoring the Founding Principles, we acknowledge that America's strength doesn't arise from fleeting trends but from enduring ideals. The rights laid down by the Founders were not given lightly; they were a gift to the future, entrusted to each new generation. Safeguarding these principles ensures that the freedoms we cherish continue to guide our national journey, nurturing a society defined by liberty, responsibility, and infinite possibility.

Embracing Free Speech as a Pillar of Liberty:

Why It Matters:

Free speech forms the backbone of a healthy and dynamic republic; allowing every voice—no matter how unpopular or unconventional—to be heard reinforces our commitment to self-governance, mutual understanding, and continuous social progress. The free exchange of ideas isn't just an abstract principle; it's how we learn, adapt, and thrive as a people. When citizens are encouraged to speak openly and listen thoughtfully, we cultivate an environment where innovation flourishes, solutions emerge, and even disagreements can pave the way toward cooperation and understanding.

Embracing free speech as a pillar of liberty means trusting Americans to debate honestly, share their perspectives, and refine their ideas through conversation. This protected and revered marketplace of ideas ensures that truth is tested rather than dictated. It challenges assumptions, sharpens arguments, and guards against stagnation when voices fall silent. In championing free speech, we affirm that progress comes not from silencing dissent but from embracing it, allowing the best ideas to take root and grow.

Guided Meditation:

Close your eyes and take three slow, steady breaths. Imagine entering a vibrant public square filled with people from all walks of life. Each person holds a different story, belief, or opinion, woven together like a colorful tapestry draped across the nation.

Walk through this square, listening to the murmurs of conversation. Some people disagree passionately, yet they keep talking, seeking common ground or greater understanding. Others exchange fresh perspectives with curiosity and respect. There are no walls here—only opportunities to learn, share, and grow.

With each breath, sense the strength born of honest debate. Feel how open dialogue lets truth shine more brightly, revealing nuances and possibilities that silence could never uncover. Recognize that by allowing all voices to speak, we protect the very principles that sustain our liberty.

Before opening your eyes, envision these conversations leading not to division but growth. Returning to the present, remember that every voice contributes to the grand American narrative. Protecting free speech ensures we continue shaping our nation's story together, guided by honesty, courage, and respect.

Affirmation: "I cherish free speech as a cornerstone of liberty, trusting that honest dialogue and respectful debate strengthen our understanding and unity."

Journaling Prompts:

Reflect on when hearing a different opinion changed or refined your perspective. How did open, respectful dialogue bring you closer to truth?

Consider what makes a marketplace of ideas healthy. How can we maintain a culture where disagreements spark growth rather than division?

Write about an issue that you care about. How might expressing your view—and listening to others—contribute to a better understanding or a more creative solution?

Practices in Action:

Engage Thoughtfully: Seek out opinions that differ from your own. Practice listening without judgment, asking questions, and considering alternative viewpoints.

Support Open Forums: Attend local debates, town halls, or community discussions. Your participation helps sustain the very spaces where free speech thrives, ensuring a more informed and empathetic citizenry.

Conclusion:

Embracing free speech as a pillar of liberty reminds us that our differences need not divide us. Instead, they can challenge us to think deeper, understand more, and emerge wiser. By defending the right to speak freely and hear others out, we uphold the ideals that the Founders entrusted to us—principles that continue to inspire growth, unity, and a brighter future for every American voice.

Protecting Religious Freedom for All:

Why It Matters:

Religious freedom isn't just a principle enshrined in our nation's founding documents; it's a living promise that allows every American to worship according to their conscience—or to choose not to worship at all. By protecting this right, we create a nation where individuals of different faiths or no faith coexist harmoniously, respecting one another's beliefs and moral compasses. Religious freedom ensures that the spiritual journey—personal, communal, or none—unfolds without fear, discrimination, or interference.

When we champion religious freedom, we celebrate the idea that America's strength comes from embracing its people's diversity. Each community's traditions, ceremonies, and ethical frameworks enrich our cultural landscape. By upholding this fundamental liberty, we encourage dialogue, understanding, and empathy across faith lines, preventing one group's beliefs from eclipsing another's. In doing so, we build a stronger, more compassionate society that honors the dignity and conscience of every individual.

Guided Meditation:

Settle into a comfortable position and close your eyes. Take three slow, steady breaths, inhaling respect and exhaling judgment. Imagine standing in a peaceful garden filled with many different flowering plants. Each bloom is unique, contributing its color, scent, and presence.

Walk through this garden, noticing that the flowers thrive side-by-side—not forced into uniformity but allowed to grow naturally as they are. Just as this garden thrives in its diversity, our nation flourishes when everyone can follow their faith tradition or choose none.

As you breathe evenly, sense the calm and mutual respect that arises when religious liberty is cherished. In this mental garden, no flower overshadows the others; each bloom adds depth and richness. This harmony reminds us that no one should feel pressured to hide or alter their beliefs to fit in in America.

Before you open your eyes, envision communities where mosques, synagogues, churches, temples, and secular gatherings coexist without fear. You carry this vision, understanding that religious freedom nurtures a culture of mutual respect, dignity, and peace.

Affirmation:

"I honor the right of every individual to follow their conscience freely, recognizing that protecting religious liberty preserves the beauty and integrity of our shared national tapestry."

Journaling Prompts:

Reflect on when you witnessed or experienced respect for differing religious or non-religious beliefs. How did that moment deepen your appreciation for religious liberty?

Consider how allowing all faiths and non-faith traditions to flourish can foster understanding and goodwill. What lessons can be drawn from this inclusiveness?

Imagine a future where religious differences are met with curiosity rather than suspicion. How might this cultural shift influence relationships, communities, and the nation?

Practices in Action:

Learn About Other Traditions: Attend community interfaith events or read about unfamiliar religious traditions. Knowledge promotes empathy and understanding, strengthening the bonds between neighbors of varying beliefs.

Speak Up for Inclusivity: When you encounter intolerance or misinformation about religious or non-religious groups, respond with patience and facts. Your voice can help create a climate of openness, ensuring everyone's freedom is respected.

Conclusion:

Protecting religious freedom for all affirms that every American's inner life and spiritual journey is their sacred ground. When we value these freedoms, we encourage respect, foster tolerance, and cultivate peaceful coexistence. In honoring religious liberty, we ensure that our nation's cultural garden continues to bloom in rich, vibrant diversity, inspiring hope and compassion in every corner of our shared home.

Defending the Right to Bear Arms:

Why It Matters:

The right to bear arms, as protected by the Second Amendment, represents more than possessing a firearm—it symbolizes personal freedom, responsibility, and the enduring American value of self-reliance. Our nation's citizens who understood this right preserved their households, communities, and sense of autonomy. The Founders intended it to safeguard against tyranny, ensuring power resides with the people rather than distant authorities.

When we defend the right to bear arms responsibly, we acknowledge that freedom is accompanied by accountability. This balance supports a society where individuals are empowered to protect themselves and their families while also respecting the rights and safety of others. By honoring the Second Amendment, we uphold a legacy of trust in the citizenry, rooted in the belief that free people, guided by principle and prudence, can maintain liberty and security.

Guided Meditation:

Find a quiet space, close your eyes, and take three calm, steady breaths. Picture yourself standing on a simple, well-worn porch overlooking vast, open land. There's a feeling of independence here—no one tells you what to believe or how to live. Instead, your freedom flourishes in harmony with the responsibility you carry.

In the distance, imagine a small homestead: sturdy walls, a family inside, and the gentle hum of a peaceful life. If ever threatened, the right to defend this home rests in your hands. Envision holding a protective and symbolic tool, reminding you that sovereignty begins at the hearth and radiates outward.

As you breathe in, sense the gravity of this freedom. It's not about fear or aggression; it's about ensuring that your well-being and neighbors are never left entirely in someone else's control. With each breath, understand that this right exists alongside compassion, good judgment, and a shared dedication to peace.

Before you open your eyes, see this vision expand: a community of informed, law-abiding citizens who value liberty and understand that strength and restraint must move hand in hand. Carry this image with you, confident that defending the right to bear arms can uphold freedom while reinforcing the bonds of trust and responsibility that hold us together.

Affirmation:

"I honor the right to bear arms as a pillar of personal freedom and responsibility, understanding that this liberty safeguards both independence and the peaceful order of our communities."

Journaling Prompts:

Reflect on what the Second Amendment means to you. How does self-reliance and responsibility shape your understanding of this right?

Consider how communities might foster a culture of respect around gun ownership. What values and practices can help maintain both safety and individual freedoms?

Envision a scenario where citizens confidently embrace their rights while prioritizing training, education, and responsible use. How might this commitment influence how we live, work, and trust one another?

Practices in Action:

Learn the Rules & Safety Measures: If you own firearms, invest time in proper training, safety courses, and regular practice. Knowledge and competence ensure that your rights serve to protect—not endanger—those around you.

Encourage Responsible Dialogue: Engage in respectful conversations about the Second Amendment, seeking common ground and understanding. You help create a community where freedom and well-being coexist by listening and learning from others.

Conclusion:

Defending the right to bear arms isn't about glorifying weapons but preserving a critical safeguard of independence and personal responsibility. In upholding this amendment, we trust one another to balance freedom with wisdom and strength with compassion. Through responsible stewardship of our rights, we continue the American tradition of self-reliance, ensuring that we remain a nation defined by liberty, dignity, and mutual respect.

Upholding Checks and Balances:

Why It Matters:

America's founders designed a system of government guided by checks and balances to prevent any branch—executive, legislative, or judicial—from growing too powerful. By distributing authority, they created a structure that safeguards our constitutional rights, ensuring that no single entity can unilaterally impose its will. This careful balance allows freedoms like free speech, religious liberty, and the right to bear arms to endure, regardless of which party or leader holds office at any given moment.

When each branch respects its constitutional role, our rights are less vulnerable to sudden shifts in policy or the ambitions of a few. Upholding checks and balances means acknowledging that enduring liberty comes not from a concentration of power but from its thoughtful division. As a result, Americans can trust that their rights remain secure and preserved under a system designed to encourage transparency, accountability, and the careful stewardship of authority.

Guided Meditation:

Close your eyes, take three deep breaths, and imagine standing in a peaceful clearing surrounded by three tall trees—each distinct yet contributing to the same vibrant ecosystem. These trees represent the three branches of government. Notice how none overshadows the others; instead, they stand in equilibrium, creating a balanced canopy of protection.

A gentle breeze rustling through their leaves symbolizes open debate and negotiation. This balanced forest thrives because power, like sunlight, is shared and not concentrated. Here, your rights find shelter under a canopy of measured governance.

With each breath, appreciate the assurance this balance provides. Just as the roots of these trees intertwine to hold the soil steady, the Constitution's checks and balances intertwine to keep our nation's foundation firm. In this environment, freedom has room to grow, unthreatened by unchecked power.

Before you open your eyes, envision future generations walking through this forest, enjoying the legacy of balanced governance. Carry this image forward, understanding that when the branches of government respect their boundaries, our constitutional rights can flourish in peace and stability.

Affirmation:

"I value the balance of power that protects our freedoms, knowing that when each branch respects its limits, our rights remain secure and enduring."

Journaling Prompts:

Reflect on why dividing power among multiple branches might help protect individual liberties. How does this structure encourage accountability and fairness?

Consider a historical event in which checks and balances were crucial. What lessons can we learn from that moment, and how do they apply to today's challenges?

Envision a future where every branch of government honors its constitutional limits. What benefits might this bring to individuals, communities, and the nation?

Practices in Action:

Stay Informed: Learn how each branch of government functions and the safeguards intended to keep them in check. An informed citizenry is better equipped to recognize when balance is threatened.

Engage Civically: Support representatives, judges, and leaders who demonstrate respect for constitutional boundaries. Your voice and your vote contribute to preserving the equilibrium that underpins our freedoms.

Conclusion:

Upholding checks and balances ensures that our constitutional rights are not dependent on the character of a single leader or party. By preserving a system where power is shared and limited, we protect the freedoms and principles that define America. Embracing this balance helps guarantee that liberty endures, allowing our nation to stand confidently on a foundation of fairness, respect, and unwavering commitment to the rights of the people.

Encouraging Civic Responsibility and Engagement:

Why It Matters:

A healthy democracy depends on the rights safeguarded by the Constitution and citizens who understand, value, and exercise those rights. When we encourage civic responsibility and engagement, we empower individuals to shape the policies and leaders that guide our nation. Informed, active participation—through voting, volunteering, attending community forums, and holding representatives accountable— ensures that the voices of everyday Americans help determine the country's direction.

Beyond casting a ballot, civic engagement builds trust, encourages cooperation, and fosters understanding among neighbors. By inspiring citizens to learn about issues, assert their constitutional liberties, and thoughtfully debate solutions, we create a society where everyone can contribute to America's ongoing story. This shared responsibility enriches our collective life, making freedom more than a concept—it becomes a vibrant, living practice.

Guided Meditation:

Close your eyes, breathe deeply three times, and imagine standing before a town hall. The lights are on inside, and you hear the soft murmur of voices. People from all walks of life have gathered, eager to listen, learn, and speak their truth.

Step inside and see individuals exchanging ideas with calm determination. They discuss local matters, national policies, and future goals. There's a hum of respect— everyone remains committed to the common good even when disagreements arise.

As you inhale, feel the strength of embracing your role as a citizen. Recognize that your voice matters, vote counts, and presence can inspire positive change. With every breath, absorb the understanding that democracy thrives when good-hearted people show up, stay informed, and engage thoughtfully.

Before opening your eyes, picture a future where generations of Americans expect to participate—knowing their rights, exercising their liberties, and contributing ideas. Carry this vision with you as you return, aware that civic responsibility is the heartbeat of a free and flourishing nation.

Affirmation:

"I actively participate in American democracy, using my knowledge, voice, and vote to preserve our freedoms and shape our shared future."

Journaling Prompts:

Reflect on a recent issue or event that motivated you to learn more, speak up, or take action. How did engaging with this topic affect your sense of empowerment?

Consider what 'good citizenship' means to you. How can understanding your constitutional rights inform how you participate in your community or nation?

Envision a more engaged, informed electorate. What steps can each individual take to make this vision a reality?

Practices in Action:

Stay Informed and speak up: Read reputable news sources, follow legislative updates, and discuss important issues with friends and family. Your informed perspective strengthens community dialogue.

Get Involved Locally: Attend a school board meeting, volunteer at a voter registration drive, or join a civic organization. Small acts of engagement at the local level help uphold the democratic process nationwide.

Conclusion:

Encouraging civic responsibility and engagement transforms abstract constitutional rights into lived experiences. When Americans assert their liberties, stay informed, and contribute their voices, they reinforce the democratic foundation laid by the Founders. In doing so, we nurture a vibrant, inclusive society where each individual's participation helps guide the nation toward a future defined by freedom, responsibility, and shared purpose.

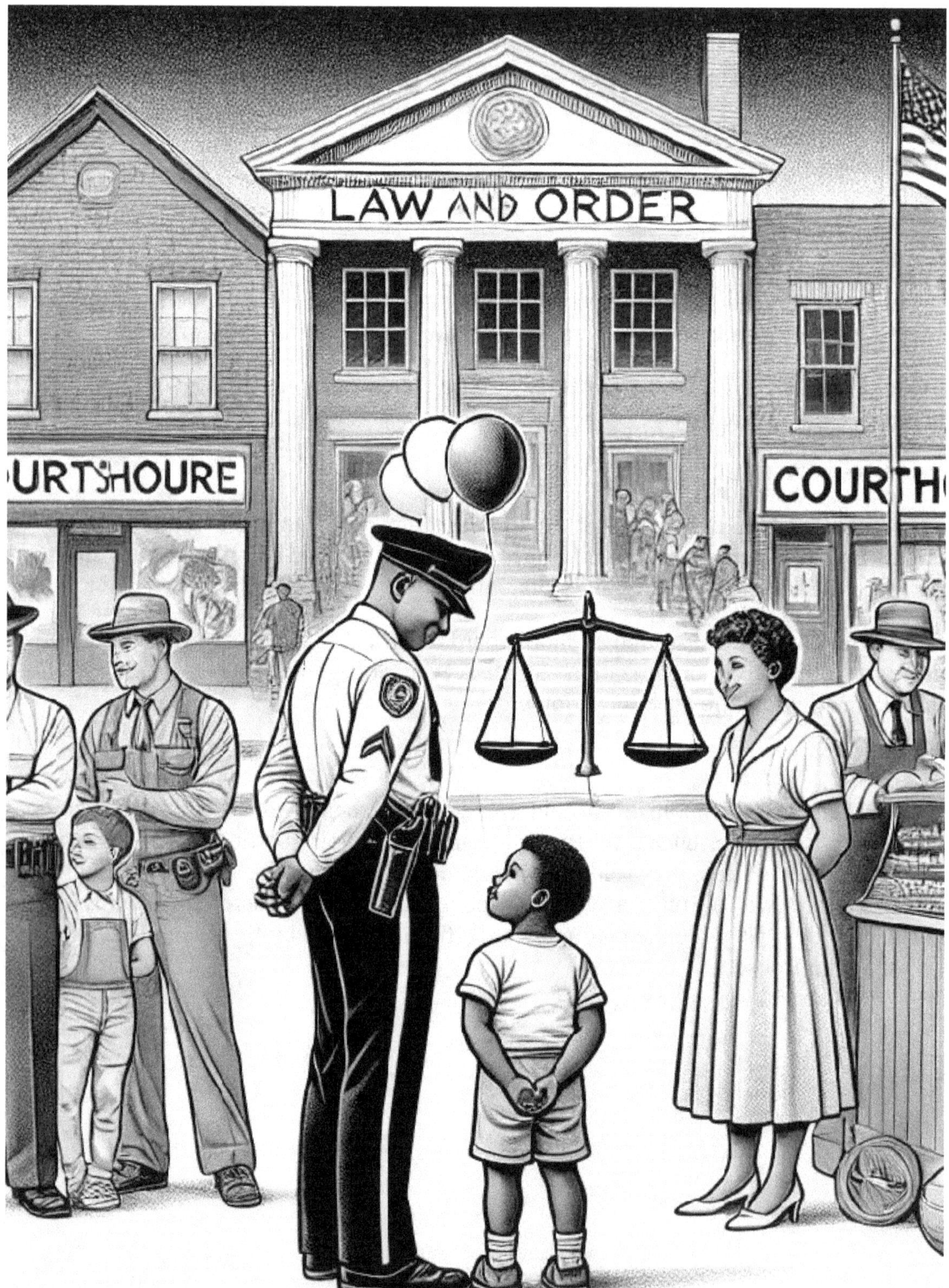

LAW AND ORDER
OURTSHOURE
COURTHO

FOUR: Law and Order

A safe and secure society is the foundation upon which individuals, families, and communities can thrive. The commitment to law and order reflects a shared belief in fairness, accountability, and the importance of protecting the vulnerable. Supporting law enforcement is about more than maintaining peace—it is about fostering trust, ensuring justice, and building communities where everyone feels secure and respected.

Police and law enforcement officers are critical in safeguarding neighborhoods and upholding the rule of law. These men and women dedicate themselves to serving their communities, often at significant personal risk. Valuing their contributions means providing the support, training, and resources they need to perform their duties effectively while fostering trust between officers and the people they serve.

A commitment to law and order includes proactive efforts to reduce crime through effective policies, community programs, and rehabilitation initiatives. Reducing crime protects individuals and strengthens the social fabric, enabling families to live without fear and businesses to flourish. True justice requires a fair, consistent system that addresses the root causes of crime while holding offenders accountable.

Public safety thrives in an environment of mutual respect and cooperation. Building trust between law enforcement and their communities is essential for effective policing. This trust is cultivated through open dialogue, transparency, and partnerships prioritizing safety and understanding. A more substantial, united society results when law enforcement and communities work together.

Movements that oppose or seek to diminish the role of law enforcement often stem from frustration and a desire for change, but they can also erode public trust and stability. Engaging in meaningful conversations about reform while opposing efforts that undermine safety ensures that progress is made without compromising security. Supporting law and order is about finding balance—promoting accountability and equity while standing firm against actions that endanger public peace.

Law and order extend beyond policing. Strong, resilient communities are built through education, economic opportunity, and programs that support youth and families. Investing in these areas reduces the conditions that lead to crime, creating environments where safety and well-being are the norm. By addressing the broader picture, we ensure that law and order are maintained and sustained through a culture of respect and care.

Valuing the Protectors of Our Communities:

Why It Matters:

Our neighborhoods, towns, and cities thrive when people feel safe and protected. Law enforcement officers dedicate their lives to this goal, often facing the unknown and putting themselves in harm's way to safeguard others. They play a vital role in maintaining peace, ensuring that families enjoy their homes, children walk to school without fear, and local businesses can serve their communities confidently.

Valuing the protectors of our communities means paying attention to the need for accountability or dialogue. Instead, it acknowledges that with the steady commitment of those who uphold the law, the very foundation of public safety would stay strong. By appreciating their dedication and sacrifices, we foster mutual respect and a willingness to work together toward safer, more secure neighborhoods.

Guided Meditation:

Close your eyes and take three gentle, steady breaths. Imagine standing on a peaceful street in your neighborhood—houses well-kept, porches bathed in warm light, and quiet voices carrying through the evening air. You feel a sense of calm and comfort in this familiar place.

As you walk along the sidewalk, picture a law enforcement officer quietly patrolling nearby, watchful and attentive. They are there not to intrude but to ensure that everyone sleeps peacefully, that children grow up unafraid, and that those who need help can find it close at hand. With each breath, recognize the courage and dedication this role requires.

Inhale, appreciating the delicate balance they maintain. Exhale, feeling gratitude for their willingness to serve. These protectors stand as a line of defense against harm, their presence enabling communities to flourish. Carry this sense of appreciation and respect with you as you open your eyes, knowing that by valuing their efforts, we support the shared goal of safety for all.

Affirmation:

"I honor the commitment of those who protect our neighborhoods, and I acknowledge their role in creating an environment where families and communities can thrive."

Journaling Prompts:

Reflect on a moment when you felt exceptionally safe or supported in your community. How might law enforcement have contributed to that sense of security?

Consider the sacrifices law enforcement officers make. How can understanding these sacrifices deepen your respect for their work and humanity?

Imagine ways to show gratitude or support for those who serve and protect. What small actions might encourage positive relationships between police and the communities they safeguard?

Practices in Action:

Reach Out and Express Thanks: When you have the opportunity, thank a local officer. Even a simple word of appreciation can strengthen community bonds.

Engage in Community Initiatives: Support or participate in programs that encourage positive dialogue between law enforcement and residents, such as neighborhood watch groups, local forums, or events that foster understanding and trust.

Conclusion:

Valuing the protectors of our communities reminds us that safety and peace aren't guaranteed—they are earned through the dedicated service of those who stand watch. By recognizing their courage, we nurture a relationship built on mutual respect, paving the way for cooperative problem-solving, stronger neighborhoods, and a stable foundation for future generations to develop their lives confidently.

Building Trust & Cooperation:

Why It Matters:

Low crime rates don't just define a thriving community; a spirit of trust and collaboration shapes it. When citizens and law enforcement officers respect one another's roles and perspectives, solving problems and finding solutions for everyone becomes easier. Mutual understanding helps break down barriers, transforming interactions from tense encounters into opportunities for support and growth.

Building trust and cooperation doesn't mean overlooking mistakes or ignoring the need for accountability. Instead, it encourages both sides to engage openly, acknowledge challenges, and seek common ground. By fostering honest communication, citizens and officers work in tandem to create neighborhoods where people feel safe, heard, and respected. This approach strengthens community bonds, ensuring that future generations inherit places defined not by division but by shared purpose and unity.

Guided Meditation:

Find a quiet, comfortable position and close your eyes. Take three slow, steady breaths. Envision yourself at a community meeting—a welcoming space filled with neighbors and local officers seated side by side. Everyone here is eager to listen and learn from one another.

Walk through the room and notice conversations taking place. People share their concerns, and officers explain their perspectives. Instead of speaking over each other, they pause, reflect, and respond with empathy. As you breathe in, feel the warmth of understanding; as you exhale, release any tension or mistrust.

Imagine these dialogues leading to meaningful change: more responsive policing, better community support, and a sense of partnership rather than opposition. With each breath, absorb the idea that honesty and compassion can mend divides, turning what once felt like distance into a bond of respect.

Before you open your eyes, picture this trust's ripple effect—families feeling safer, neighborhoods growing more assertive, and local traditions thriving. Carry this image with you, knowing that cooperation is a powerful force for shaping communities that uplift everyone.

Affirmation:

"I encourage respectful, honest communication between law enforcement and citizens, knowing that trust and cooperation strengthen the fabric of our communities."

Journaling Prompts:

Reflect on how understanding another person's perspective improves a situation. How can this principle apply to building trust between police and neighbors?

Consider what steps might help bridge gaps in your community—more open meetings, shared events, or educational forums. How could you contribute to fostering these interactions?

Envision a future where cooperation, not conflict, defines the relationship between law enforcement and citizens. What positive changes emerge in that scenario?

Practices in Action:

Attend Community-Police Dialogues: If your area hosts forums, panels, or workshops bringing residents and officers together, consider participating. Your presence and input help nourish constructive dialogue.

Promote Understanding Through Education: Encourage local schools, community centers, or religious organizations to host events or classes that highlight the roles, challenges, and experiences of both citizens and law enforcement.

Conclusion:

Building trust and cooperation between law enforcement and citizens lays the groundwork for healthier, more united neighborhoods. Fear and suspicion yield to understanding and partnership when both sides communicate openly and respectfully. In this environment, individuals, families, and entire communities experience a newfound sense of security, optimism, and connectedness—growing ever more potent as they move together.

Ensuring Safe Streets & Neighborhoods:

Why It Matters:

Safe streets and neighborhoods are the foundation upon which families build their futures, children discover their potential, and local businesses take root. When crime rates decline and public safety improves, communities experience a ripple effect of positive outcomes: schools can focus more on education than security, small businesses gain loyal customers, and neighbors feel comfortable venturing out to support local events. Strong, stable neighborhoods empower people to invest their time, energy, and creativity in the places they call home.

Ensuring everyone feels secure fosters an environment where opportunity thrives and hope flourishes. Improved public safety isn't just about preventing harm; it's about nurturing a shared sense of belonging that encourages individuals to contribute their talents, protect their neighbors, and celebrate their shared values. In nurturing safer communities, we create a brighter future for everyone there.

Guided Meditation:

Find a calm, quiet space and close your eyes. Take three steady breaths, envisioning a neighborhood street bathed in gentle evening light. Laughter drifts from a nearby porch, and children's bicycles rest safely at the curb.

Picture parents walking with their children, unhurried and relaxed. Imagine storefronts open late, their warm lights inviting passersby to step inside. As you breathe in, feel the calm assurance that people care for each other's well-being. With each exhalation, let go of any lingering fears or anxieties.

Since the collective effort that maintains this peace. Law enforcement officers who uphold the law responsibly, neighbors who watch out for one another, and local leaders who prioritize community safety. Each breath connects you more deeply to the idea that these conditions are not accidental but earned through respect, cooperation, and vigilance.

Hold onto the image of this peaceful street before opening your eyes. Carry this vision with you, knowing that ensuring public safety isn't just about reducing crime; it's about making room for families, friendships, creativity, and everyday joys to flourish in the open air.

Affirmation:

"I recognize that secure neighborhoods nurture stronger families, growing children, and thriving local businesses, and I support efforts that sustain this peaceful foundation."

Journaling Prompts:

Reflect on when you felt genuinely safe in your community. What made that environment possible, and how did it impact your well-being?

Consider how reduced crime affects individuals and local economies. What benefits might arise when businesses can operate without fear and neighbors trust one another implicitly?

Envision changes that could improve safety where you live—better street lighting, neighborhood watch programs, or youth engagement activities. How could you contribute to bringing these improvements to life?

Practices in Action:

Support Local Initiatives: Volunteer with or donate to community groups focused on crime prevention, youth mentorship, or neighborhood revitalization. Your involvement helps sustain conditions that keep families safe and engaged.

Practice Vigilant Neighborliness: Monitor your surroundings and offer support when something seems off. This everyday watchfulness strengthens trust among residents and reinforces the notion that everyone plays a role in public safety.

Conclusion:

Ensuring safe streets and neighborhoods goes beyond statistics—it shapes our daily experiences, long-term aspirations, and the paths our children will travel. When communities commit to reducing crime and fostering security, they open doors to prosperity, unity, and optimism. In doing so, they transform ordinary blocks into places where relationships deepen, opportunities abound, and the promise of a better life is available to all.

Reinforcing Respect for the Rule of Law:

Why It Matters:

A society built on fairness, consistency, and justice stands firm against the currents of uncertainty and mistrust. When the rule of law is upheld with integrity, individuals know their rights are protected, their voices are heard, and no one stands above the standards agreed upon by all. This foundation protects everyone's liberty, ensuring people can speak, worship, and engage in daily life without fearing arbitrary actions.

By reinforcing respect for the rule of law, we guard against corruption and abuse of power and promote greater harmony within our communities. Fair, consistent enforcement weaves a sense of security and belonging into the social fabric, encouraging citizens to trust their institutions. In this environment, cooperation and mutual respect flourish, allowing American ideals to thrive and strengthening the bonds that unite us as a people.

Guided Meditation:

Close your eyes and take three calm breaths. Imagine standing in a peaceful town square framed by well-tended buildings. In this space, people move freely, confident that their rights are upheld and protected.

Picture a statue at the center of the square, representing the rule of law—its expression serene, its posture steady. As you inhale, feel the stability it imparts; as you exhale, let go of any doubt. Here, fairness is not a distant ideal but a daily reality.

Observe neighbors exchanging greetings, local leaders listening attentively to concerns, and law enforcement officers quietly reassuring with their presence. Each breath reminds you that liberty and order coexist harmoniously when rules are clear and applied.

Before you open your eyes, carry this image with you: a community bound by trust and shared purpose, where justice is spoken of and lived daily.

Affirmation:

"I uphold the principles of fairness and integrity, knowing that respect for the rule of law preserves freedom, strengthens communities, and enriches our shared future."

Journaling Prompts:

Recall a time when knowing your rights and the laws that protect them brought you comfort or clarity. What did that experience teach you about the value of a just system?

Consider how fairness and consistency in law enforcement build trust between citizens and authorities. What positive outcomes might arise from this mutual respect?

Envision a scenario where every community member feels seen, heard, and treated equally under the law. How could this shape how people interact, cooperate, and care for one another?

Practices in Action:

Educate Yourself: Learn about local and national laws that affect your community. Understanding these laws ensures you can advocate for fairness and hold leaders accountable when necessary.

Support Fair Legal Processes: Encourage or participate in programs that promote transparency, such as community police boards, town hall meetings, or local forums. By staying involved, you help safeguard the standards that protect individual liberties.

Conclusion:

Respect for the rule of law reinforces the American promise that no one is above justice and that every person can count on fairness and consistency. By embracing these principles, we nurture an environment where freedom and security reinforce one another. This balanced approach to governance ensures that our freedoms endure, our communities remain vibrant, and the fundamental dignity of every individual is honored.

Encouraging Civic Responsibility:

Why It Matters:

Proper security and stability in our communities depend on law enforcement's efforts and engaged citizens' active participation. When individuals take responsibility for their neighborhoods—reporting suspicious activities, mentoring youth, and maintaining respectful public discourse—they help create environments where crime struggles to gain a foothold. Embracing personal accountability acknowledges that each of us has a role in keeping our streets safe and nurturing a sense of shared ownership over the places we call home.

Encouraging civic responsibility fosters cooperation between residents and those who enforce the law. This partnership generates trust and understanding, making preventing problems before they escalate easier. When citizens step up to support their local communities, they send a powerful message: we're in this together, committed to ensuring that our towns and cities remain welcoming havens of stability, opportunity, and pride.

Guided Meditation:

Find a quiet, comfortable space and close your eyes. Inhale slowly, picturing a familiar neighborhood street. Imagine seeing neighbors waving hello, parents chatting as children play, and local officers patrolling calmly, ready to help.

Walk down this street in your mind's eye. Notice how everyone contributes in their own way—a teen keeping the park clean, a shopkeeper who knows every customer's name, a resident who volunteers at a community watch program. With each breath, sense the collective energy generated by people who care.

As you inhale, feel the strength from knowing you're part of this whole. Exhale any doubts that your actions matter. In this vision, each person's effort, big or small, maintains the balance that allows everyone to flourish.

Before you open your eyes, envision yourself taking action that supports your community—speaking kindly to a neighbor, volunteering for a local cause, or simply staying informed. Carry this intention with you as you return to the present, knowing you can help maintain order and safety.

Affirmation:

"I embrace my responsibility to support my community, cooperate with law enforcement, and uphold the shared values that keep our neighborhoods secure and welcoming."

Journaling Prompts:

Reflect on a time when you took action—no matter how small—to improve safety or harmony in your community. How did it feel to know you made a difference?

Consider how civic responsibility and personal accountability strengthen trust between citizens and police. How might this trust impact the future of your neighborhood?

Envision a community where everyone takes ownership of maintaining order. What changes would you see in how people interact, solve problems, and celebrate successes?

Practices in Action:

Get Involved Locally: Volunteer for a neighborhood watch program, help organize a community clean-up or attend local safety meetings. Your participation encourages others to follow suit.

Be a Good Neighbor: Learn your neighbors' names, listen to their concerns, and work together on mutual goals. Small acts of kindness and cooperation form the building blocks of a safer, more unified community.

Conclusion:

Encouraging civic responsibility recognizes that safety and harmony don't come solely from the top down—they grow from the ground up, rooted in everyday citizens who care. By working alongside law enforcement, respecting one another, and holding ourselves accountable, we weave a resilient social fabric. In doing so, we ensure that the ideals of order and stability are not just principles but lived realities in the places we cherish.

Challenging Anti-Authority Narratives:

Why It Matters:

When trust in our institutions is eroded by anti-authority narratives, the framework that ensures safety and harmony weakens. These narratives can sow division, encouraging individuals to view law enforcement and other authority figures as inherently oppressive rather than as essential partners in upholding peace and justice. Such a perspective threatens to undo the delicate balance that allows free societies to function—where checks and balances protect our liberties, and enforcement ensures fairness and security for all.

Challenging anti-authority narratives doesn't mean disregarding legitimate concerns or refusing honest dialogue. Instead, it involves recognizing that dismissing all authority can fracture communities, discourage collaboration, and ultimately harm the most vulnerable. By pushing back against these damaging outlooks, we nurture a culture of respect, cooperation, and shared purpose. In doing so, we strengthen the values that have long anchored our nation's prosperity and ensured that safety and freedom flourish.

Guided Meditation:

Close your eyes, take three deep breaths, and picture yourself on a well-trodden path through a peaceful park. You see families strolling, friends laughing, and neighbors nodding hello as they pass by. This sense of calm and connection is possible because everyone respects specific rules and trusts the system that protects them.

Imagine a sudden whisper moving through the crowd that authority cannot be trusted. See how people become wary, distant, and guarded. The easy smiles fade, replaced by suspicion. Notice how this negativity seems to cast a shadow over the once-bright landscape.

Breathe slowly, and as you exhale, envision yourself gently pushing back the shadow, bringing in light that reminds everyone of the value of working together. With each breath, reaffirm that fair authority and respectful dialogue hold communities together, preventing chaos and harm.

Before you open your eyes, see the park returning to its vibrant warmth. People are more willing to listen, more eager to cooperate, and more ready to uphold the values that secure their shared space. Carry this vision with you; knowing your understanding can help keep anti-authority narratives in check.

Affirmation:

"I reject narratives that undermine trust and stability, choosing instead to support balanced authority and cooperation that safeguard our shared prosperity."

Journaling Prompts:

Recall when trust in an institution brings reassurance or stability to your life. How did that sense of trust improve your experiences?

Consider the long-term impact of widespread mistrust. How might anti-authority sentiments, when left unchecked, reshape neighborhoods, schools, or civic life?

Envision steps you might take to encourage balanced discussions about authority figures. How can you help friends or neighbors understand the difference between healthy skepticism and harmful cynicism?

Practices in Action:

Participate in Dialogue: Join local forums or community discussions focused on issues of authority and justice. Your perspective can help counter sweeping anti-authority sentiments with reasoned, empathetic understanding.

Highlight Positive Examples: Share stories of law enforcement and community leaders collaborating effectively. Reminding others of these positive partnerships reinforces that trust and authority can—and often do—work hand in hand.

Conclusion:

Challenging anti-authority narratives protects the societal framework that enables communities to prosper. By distinguishing between constructive critique and broad distrust, we uphold the ideals of cooperation, fairness, and security that define a healthy democracy. In doing so, we ensure that the cornerstone values of our nation—stability, liberty, and mutual respect—remain firmly in place for generations to come.

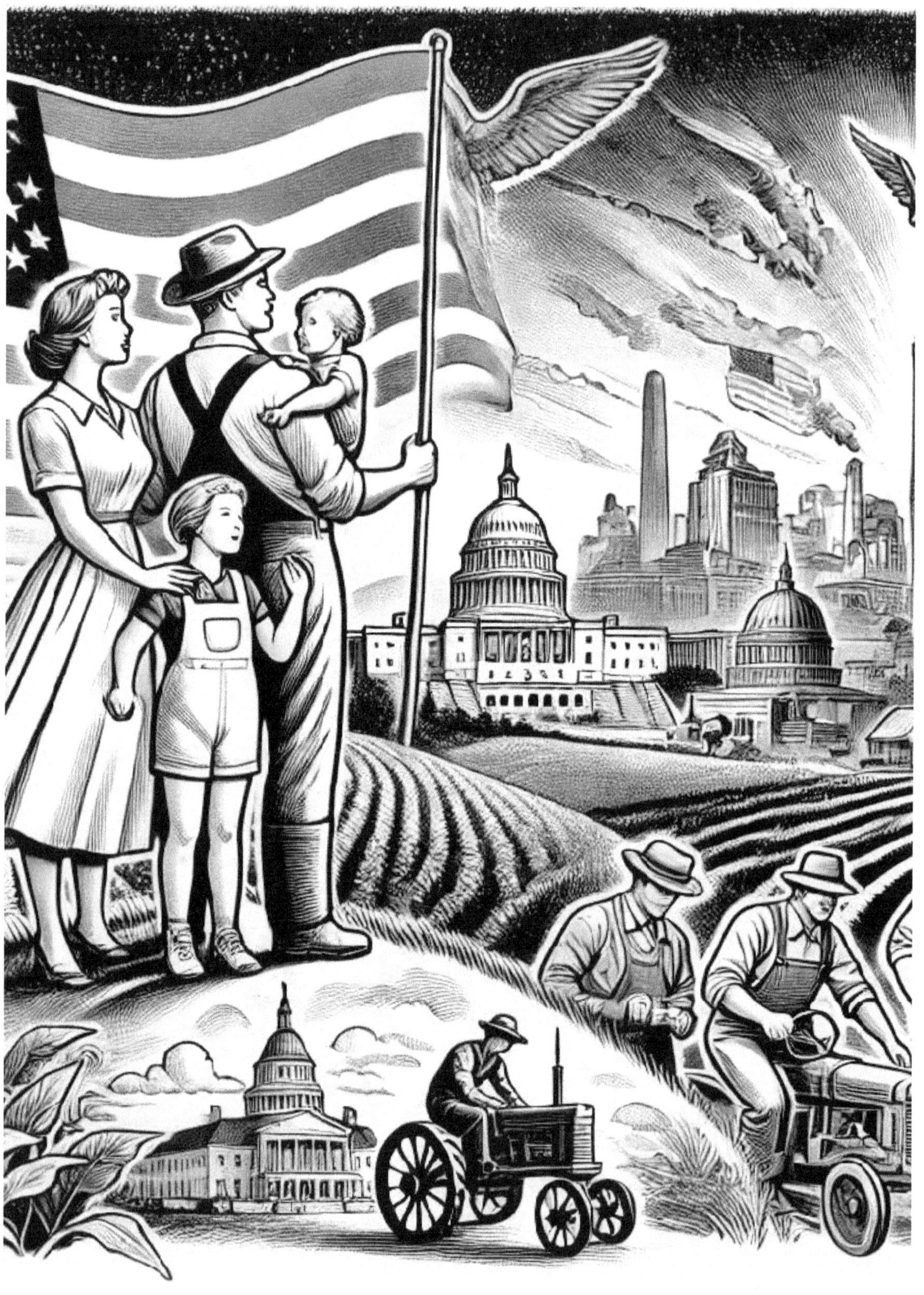

FIVE: Patriotism and National Sovereignty

Patriotism is the heartfelt appreciation of a nation's history, culture, and values. For Americans, it is a celebration of the principles of liberty, independence, and opportunity that have defined the nation since its founding. National sovereignty, meanwhile, ensures that these values are preserved by maintaining the right of self-determination and protecting the interests of the American people. Together, patriotism and sovereignty form the backbone of a proud, resilient nation.

American history is a tapestry of triumphs, challenges, and progress. Celebrating this heritage is about honoring the sacrifices and achievements of those who built the nation and reflecting on the lessons of the past to guide the future. Patriotism thrives in communities where diverse cultures and traditions are embraced as part of the larger American story. By cherishing history and culture, we strengthen the ties that unite us and inspire future generations to contribute to the legacy of this great nation.

National sovereignty is the principle that a country's people should make decisions free from undue influence by outside forces. This independence allows the United States to uphold its values, protect its citizens, and determine its path forward. Preserving sovereignty means advocating for policies prioritizing American interests and ensuring that cooperation with other nations never comes at the expense of self-reliance or autonomy.

While global collaboration can address shared challenges, unchecked globalist agendas risk diluting individual nations' unique identities and interests. Patriotism calls for mindful engagement with the international community, safeguarding national sovereignty while contributing responsibly to global efforts. By protecting America's independence, we ensure that the nation's voice remains strong and its values remain intact.

Patriotism is not about exclusion—it is about inclusion, celebrating the shared values and traditions that unite Americans while respecting the diverse backgrounds that enrich the nation. When we foster pride in our country, we create a sense of belonging that strengthens communities and inspires collaboration. By teaching younger generations about the nation's history and ideals, we ensure that the spirit of patriotism endures and evolves with time.

Patriotism and national sovereignty are forward-looking values. They remind us of the importance of protecting freedom, nurturing innovation, and pursuing progress while staying true to the principles that define us. By celebrating the past and protecting the present, we create a future where the United States remains a beacon of hope, opportunity, and strength for future generations.

Honoring American Heritage & Traditions:

Why It Matters:

The American story is a tapestry woven from countless threads—triumphs and challenges, sacrifices and breakthroughs, traditions and ideals. Each generation has contributed its chapter, passing on values like courage, independence, and hard work. By honoring American heritage and traditions, we acknowledge that who we are today is shaped by those who came before us. These stories and legacies give us a sense of rootedness, continuity, and gratitude for the struggles and successes that paved our way.

Celebrating our heritage doesn't mean disregarding past imperfections; it means learning from them and carrying forward the virtues that still ring true. Recognizing the resilience, creativity, and moral conviction passed down through the ages can inspire us to uphold cherished customs, embrace meaningful change, and work together to keep America a place of opportunity, freedom, and pride.

Guided Meditation:

Find a quiet place, close your eyes, and take three steady breaths. Imagine yourself standing before a grand, old quilt, each patch representing an era of American history—some bright and celebratory, others darker and worn, but all essential to the whole.

Move closer and notice the details on each piece of fabric: a handwritten letter from a pioneer, a newspaper clipping announcing a great invention, or an old photograph capturing a family's journey. With each breath, feel the weight of these joyful and challenging stories and sense the courage, hope, and determination that thread them together.

Imagine gently running your hand over the quilt, absorbing its warmth. Each generation's achievements, sacrifices, and traditions flow into you, guiding your understanding of who we are and how far we've come. Let these insights ground you, connecting your heart with the nation's soul.

Before you open your eyes, envision passing this quilt on to someone younger, offering them the wisdom and strength woven into every stitch. As you return to the present, carry this appreciation for American heritage, confident you can honor the past while working to create a brighter future.

Affirmation:

"I cherish the legacy passed down through generations, honoring the traditions and values that shape America's proud identity."

Journaling Prompts:

Reflect on a family tradition, local custom, or national holiday with special meaning. What values does it represent, and why do they matter today?

Learning about American history—its triumphs and trials—can inform how you contribute to society. What lessons can you apply to your own life?

Envision sharing a piece of American heritage—a story, a recipe, or a historical anecdote—with future generations. What do you hope they gain from it?

Practices in Action:

Learn & Share: Read a biography of a historic American figure, watch a documentary, or visit a museum. Share what you learn with friends and family to keep these stories alive.

Participate in Local Traditions: Attend community celebrations, festivals, or commemorations that honor America's heritage. Your presence and curiosity help sustain cherished customs.

Conclusion:
Honoring American heritage and traditions invites us to stand on the shoulders of those who came before us, drawing strength from their perseverance, innovation, and moral conviction. By appreciating this legacy, we understand the values that have guided America's journey and continue to shape its future. With respect for our past and hope for tomorrow, we reaffirm our identity as a nation defined by resilience, unity, and enduring promise.

Celebrating the Symbols of Freedom:

Why It Matters:

Symbols like the American flag, national monuments, and cultural landmarks are potent reminders of who we are and what we value. These symbols aren't just decorations; they're stories told in stone, fabric, and tradition. They resonate across generations, reminding us of shared struggles and achievements and inspiring us to carry those lessons forward. By celebrating these symbols of freedom, we strengthen the ties that bind us as one people, united in purpose and hopeful about the future.

Cherishing these icons doesn't mean ignoring the complexity of our past. It means acknowledging that, despite differences and debates, we hold ideals in common—liberty, justice, and opportunity. These shared principles give the flag its meaning, enrich the messages carried by our monuments, and illuminate our cultural landmarks. In honoring these symbols, we reaffirm the unity and resilience at the heart of the American experience.

Guided Meditation:

Close your eyes and take three even breaths. Imagine standing before a towering monument etched with words of hope, bravery, and sacrifice. Feel the quiet hush in the air, as if generations of voices have gathered here to be heard and remembered.

Slowly shift your gaze to a flag gently waving nearby. The sunlight passes through its colors, brightening reds, whites, and blues that speak of freedom and responsibility. Inhale deeply, absorbing the courage and convictions represented in those patterns of stars and stripes.

Envision other landmarks—museums, historic buildings, and cultural festivals—each telling a chapter of the American story. With every breath, sense a deeper connection to your fellow citizens, past and present, finding meaning in these shared symbols.

Before opening your eyes, imagine returning home with a renewed appreciation for these symbols' common ideals. Feel the steady assurance that celebrating these icons strengthens the unity and purpose that define our nation.

Affirmation:

"I honor the flag, monuments, and cultural landmarks as enduring symbols of freedom that unite us, remind us of our shared values, and guide us forward."

Journaling Prompts:

Think of a national symbol or landmark that resonates with you. Why does it speak to you, and what message do you take from it?

Reflect on how these symbols inspire unity. How might they help bridge differences and remind us that we share a common identity?

Envision introducing someone from another country to these American symbols. What would you highlight, and what would you hope they understand about our nation?

Practices in Action:

Learn the Stories Behind the Symbols: Read about the flag's history, the monument's creation, or the origins of a cultural landmark. Understanding their roots deepens your appreciation for their meaning.

Visit & Share: If possible, visit a monument or museum commemorating American ideals. Take a friend or family member and discuss what you learn, ensuring these symbols continue to educate and inspire.

Conclusion:

By celebrating the symbols of freedom, we recognize the threads that connect us and our past. These flags, monuments, and landmarks aren't static relics—they live in our hearts and minds, continually renewing our sense of purpose as a people. In cherishing them, we strengthen the bonds of unity and remind ourselves that the shared aspiration for liberty and understanding endures beyond every challenge.

Embracing the Spirit of Independence:

Why It Matters

At the heart of America's founding lies a profound belief in self-governance—the idea that power should originate with the people and not be granted by distant authorities. Embracing the spirit of independence means celebrating the freedoms that allow individuals to make their own choices, shape their communities, and determine their futures. This outlook values personal responsibility and collective resilience, recognizing that liberty thrives when citizens understand their role in guiding the destiny of their nation.

By cherishing independence, we acknowledge that every voice matters, every dream can ignite change, and every initiative can leave a meaningful imprint. The American story is one of charting our course, not waiting for permission from elsewhere. When we embrace this spirit, we ensure that our society remains dynamic, creative, and engaged, always moving forward with confidence and conviction.

Guided Meditation:

Close your eyes, taking three steady breaths. Imagine a broad landscape—wide-open fields under a clear sky. Feel the gentle breeze as you stand free and unencumbered, knowing you can choose your path, beliefs, and pursuits.

Imagine walking across this vast space, each step echoing self-governance principles. You determine your direction and pace, inspired by the understanding that your decisions shape your reality. With every breath, feel the strength of owning your choices and the opportunities that arise from forging your way.

Inhale the confidence of a people who value independence, trusting that innovation and progress are born when citizens take the initiative rather than await instructions. Exhale any doubts, and acknowledge the quiet assurance that comes from knowing you are not bound by limits imposed from afar.

Before you open your eyes, envision a thriving community flourishing within this open space—families, neighbors, and leaders working together, guided by mutual respect and free will. Carry this vision with you, proud to embrace the spirit of independence that empowers us all.

Affirmation:

"I celebrate the spirit of independence, honoring the freedom and responsibility that allow Americans to shape their destiny and govern themselves."

Journaling Prompts:

Reflect on a time you made an important decision without outside pressure. How did exercising personal choice and responsibility impact your sense of independence?

Consider the relationship between individual freedoms and community well-being. How can the exercise of personal liberty contribute to the greater good?

Envision what America looks like when citizens fully embrace self-governance. What changes, improvements, or innovations might emerge?

Practices in Action:

Get Involved Locally: Exercise independence by attending town hall meetings, joining a community group, or volunteering. Your engagement at the grassroots level strengthens self-governance.

Support Entrepreneurship: Encourage and patronize small businesses and startups. Their existence reflects the spirit of self-determination, proving that individuals charting their path can fuel local prosperity.

Conclusion:

Embracing the spirit of independence nurtures a society where individuals are not mere observers but active participants in shaping the world around them. By celebrating this core principle, we honor the founding idea that Americans hold the power to direct their own lives, steer their communities, and chart a future defined by freedom, creativity, and collective strength.

Preserving Cultural Pride & Diversity:

Why It Matters:

American culture is a mosaic formed by countless pieces—different heritages, faiths, traditions, and stories that have found a home within our nation's borders. Preserving cultural pride and diversity means recognizing that patriotism isn't confined to one lineage or worldview. Instead, it thrives in the richness of multiple voices, the blending of new ideas, and the wisdom passed down through generations from every corner of the globe. By celebrating this tapestry, we embrace the truth that our strength lies not in uniformity but in the harmony created by genuine respect for differences.

Valuing diversity within our sense of national pride encourages understanding, empathy, and cooperation. It acknowledges that each community's journey adds texture to our collective narrative. Rather than diluting what makes us unique, our shared patriotism magnifies these cultural notes, weaving them into a symphony of perspectives and experiences. In doing so, we honor the many threads that form the fabric of one resilient, evolving, and inclusive American family.

Guided Meditation:

Close your eyes and take three slow, steady breaths. Envision stands in a sunlit meadow surrounded by people of varied backgrounds, each wearing garments decorated with symbols of their culture. Hear the soft hum of multiple languages, each voice contributing its melody.

As you breathe in, feel gratitude for the richness different traditions bring to our shores. See neighbors passing foods with ancestral flavors and friends sharing stories stretching back decades or centuries. Allow yourself to sense the warmth and familiarity that grow when we acknowledge each other's histories.

Inhale slowly, letting the vibrant tapestry of customs and beliefs fill you with appreciation. Exhale any notion that patriotism must be one-dimensional. Instead, picture pride that welcomes all voices to the table.

Before opening your eyes, imagine these diverse communities dancing together in a circle, each step in rhythm despite distinct styles and tempos. Carry this vision with you, understanding that our shared patriotism gains depth and meaning when enriched by the variety of who we are.

Affirmation:

"I celebrate the vibrant array of cultures that unite us, understanding that true patriotism embraces the diversity that makes America strong and whole."

Journaling Prompts:

Reflect on a cultural tradition, holiday, or practice you've learned from someone outside your background. How has it broadened your perspective?

Consider how diversity strengthens our communities—through food, art, religion, language, and more. What do we gain when we honor these differences?

Envision a future where every new generation cherishes America's cultural mosaic. How might this inclusive patriotism shape the nation's identity?

Practices in Action:

Learn From Others: Attend cultural fairs, visit ethnic museums, or try dishes from various culinary traditions. By actively seeking to understand different backgrounds, you reinforce the bonds that tie us together.

Support Multicultural Initiatives: Volunteer for community programs or educational workshops celebrating heritage and customs. Helping to preserve these stories ensures they continue to enrich our national tapestry.

Conclusion:

Preserving cultural pride and diversity reaffirms that America's greatness isn't defined by a single narrative but by a chorus of voices. When we embrace each other's stories, beliefs, and traditions, we build bridges of empathy and understanding. In honoring all the cultural threads that make up our national fabric, we affirm a patriotism that thrives on unity in difference, ensuring that the American family grows ever more assertive, inclusive, and deeply connected.

Guarding Against Globalist Overreach:

Why It Matters:

While building relationships with other countries can lead to greater prosperity, safety, and innovation, international cooperation must respect America's sovereignty. Guarding against globalist overreach means ensuring that partnerships with foreign powers do not erode the nation's ability to set its policies, protect its citizens, and chart its path. Instead of relinquishing control to distant organizations or external agendas, America should engage with the world from a position of strength and principle.

This approach doesn't reject globalization—instead, it calls for balanced collaboration that prioritizes national interests and the well-being of American families. By confidently navigating global challenges, America can remain a positive force internationally, offering friendship and alliance on terms that do not compromise its independence or security. Upholding this balance safeguards the freedoms, opportunities, and self-determination that define the American way of life.

Guided Meditation:

Close your eyes, take three relaxed breaths, and visualize yourself standing at a point where two roads meet. One path leads to productive, respectful partnerships with other nations, while the other risks entanglements that diminish American independence.

Imagine walking the balanced path—the vibrant landscape has strong industries, secure borders, and a confident population. You see international neighbors extending a hand in friendship. Each partnership is rooted in mutual benefit and respect, not surrendering key decisions to outside interests.

With every breath, feel assured that while America can help shape a better world, it must not abandon its principles or sovereignty. Inhale the understanding that genuine cooperation doesn't require losing oneself; exhale any fears that looking outward must mean weakening what lies within.

Before you open your eyes, picture the American flag waving proudly overhead, a reminder that engaging globally should strengthen, not undermine, the nation's core values. Carry this vision with you, knowing that a balanced approach to international relations preserves security and freedom.

Affirmation:

"I value cooperation with other nations, always ensuring that our engagement strengthens America's sovereignty, self-reliance, and guiding principles."

Journaling Prompts:

Reflect on what sovereignty means to you. How does maintaining self-determination benefit the everyday lives of Americans?

Consider how international cooperation can uplift the United States and other nations without compromising American independence. What does balanced engagement look like?

Imagine future economic, environmental, and technological challenges where global cooperation might be necessary. How can America lead effectively while preserving its autonomy?

Practices in Action:

Stay Informed About International Agreements: Learn about trade deals, defense pacts, and global initiatives that affect the United States. Understanding these relationships helps you advocate for balanced solutions.

Engage in Civic Dialogue: Discuss with friends and neighbors how America can collaborate internationally without sacrificing its interests. Thoughtful conversation encourages policies that strike the right balance between global engagement and sovereign self-determination.

Conclusion:

Guarding against globalist overreach ensures that America's voice remains strong and independent in an interconnected world. By entering into alliances and agreements without compromising the nation's foundational values, Americans safeguard the freedom, prosperity, and security that have long defined their way of life. In doing so, they affirm that true strength lies in guiding their destiny, even as they work alongside others toward a brighter global future.

Passing the Torch of Patriotism:

Why It Matters:

Patriotism is not static—it grows, adapts, and finds new expression as each generation adds its voice to the American story. Passing the torch of patriotism means encouraging young people to embrace the values, traditions, and freedoms that form our national identity while inspiring them to shape these ideals for the challenges of tomorrow. By nurturing respect for what we've inherited and empowering youth to contribute their perspectives, we ensure that the love of the country doesn't fade but becomes more meaningful over time.

When we guide younger generations to honor the past, engage in the present, and envision the future, we help them recognize that patriotism involves gratitude and responsibility. It's about caring enough to preserve what's good and courageous enough to improve what needs changing. Through their informed dedication, the ideals of liberty, opportunity, and unity can thrive for centuries.

Guided Meditation:

Close your eyes and take three deep breaths. Picture yourself standing in a place representing America's heritage—a quiet library with historical documents or a family gathering where stories are shared.

Imagine a younger individual beside you—a child, a teenager, or a curious young adult. You offer them a small, shining torch, symbolizing the knowledge and love of country that you carry. They accept it, eyes bright with possibility.

With each breath, sense a bridge forming between the past and the future. You feel the strength of ancestors who built the foundations of freedom, and you see the promise of new generations who will interpret and uphold those ideals in their own way.

Before you open your eyes, envision this young person stepping forward, proudly holding the torch, prepared to bring patriotism into a future they will help define. Carry this hope with you, confident that by fostering pride and responsibility, America's best qualities will endure.

Affirmation:

"I trust younger generations to embrace our nation's values, shape its future, and carry the torch of patriotism forward with integrity and purpose."

Journaling Prompts:

Recall when someone shared a piece of American history or tradition with you. How did it influence your understanding of patriotism?

Consider ways to inspire younger people—through storytelling, mentorship, or education—to appreciate their country's heritage. What impact could these efforts have on the nation's future?

Envision a more inclusive, forward-looking patriotism that resonates with the challenges and opportunities ahead. How can passing the torch encourage adaptation without losing sight of fundamental principles?

Practices in Action:

Share Stories & Traditions: Spend time talking with younger family members or community youth about America's past, explaining the meaning behind holidays, monuments, and cultural practices.

Encourage Civic Engagement: Help young adults register to vote, volunteer in their communities, or join local organizations. By actively participating, they learn that patriotism flourishes when individuals take responsibility for shaping their nation's trajectory.

Conclusion:

Passing the torch of patriotism ensures that the love of the country is not merely remembered but actively lived. By connecting generations through shared values and guiding principles, we keep America's story unfolding, each chapter enriched by fresh voices and perspectives. In this exchange of wisdom and aspiration, patriotism remains a vibrant, evolving force that honors the past, embraces the present, and invests in a future guided by the strength and vision of those who come next.

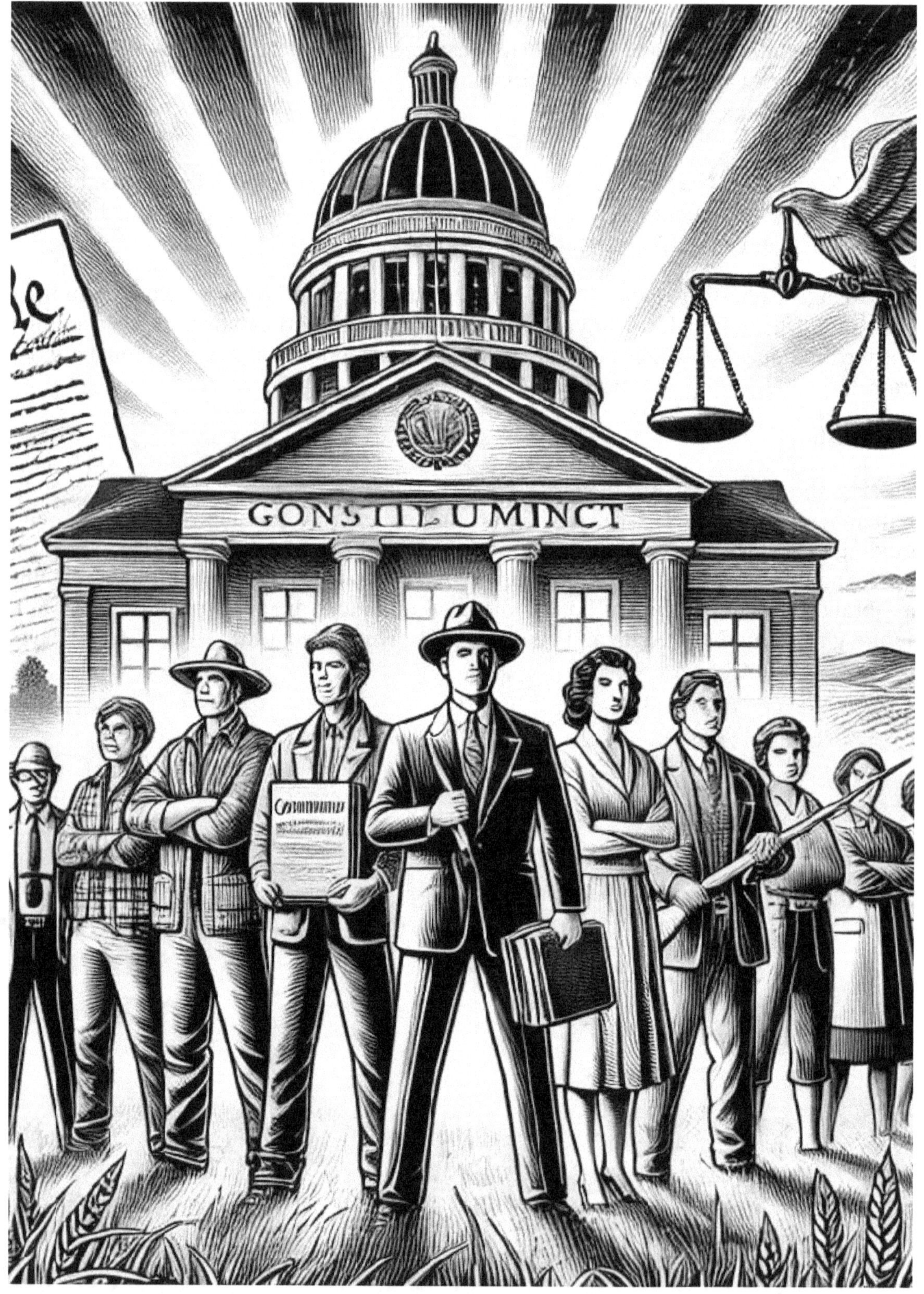
GONSTL UMINCT

SIX: Opposition to Government Overreach

Freedom is the cornerstone of the American identity, and preserving that freedom requires vigilance against excessive government overreach. When regulations, mandates, or centralized decision-making become overly burdensome, they can stifle innovation, erode personal autonomy, and limit the ability of communities and states to govern themselves effectively. Opposition to government overreach is not about rejecting governance—it is about ensuring that power remains balanced and that individual and community rights are respected.

At its core, opposition to overreach is about affirming the right of individuals to make decisions about their lives. Excessive regulations can interfere with everything from healthcare choices to how businesses operate, imposing unnecessary obstacles and limiting opportunity. Respecting personal freedom means trusting people to make decisions for themselves and their families while providing a system that supports—not restricts—their ability to thrive.

Decentralized power is a defining feature of American governance, allowing states and localities to address issues that reflect their unique needs and values. When centralized control encroaches on state or community authority, it can undermine the principle of self-governance. Empowering states and local governments ensures that decisions are made closer to the people they affect, fostering practical solutions and reflecting regional priorities.

Excessive bureaucracy can lead to inefficiency and waste, diverting resources from meaningful action. Layers of red tape often create unnecessary delays, complicate simple processes, and make it harder for individuals and businesses to navigate systems. Challenging bureaucratic expansion means advocating for streamlined governance that is transparent, accountable, and focused on serving the public effectively.

A government that respects its limits remains accountable to its people. Transparency in decision-making builds trust, ensuring that policies are driven by the public good rather than special interests or political agendas. By demanding accountability, citizens reaffirm their role as active participants in governance, helping to shape a system that works for everyone.

Limiting government overreach empowers individuals and communities to take responsibility for their success and well-being. Self-reliance fosters innovation, strengthens families, and builds resilience, creating a society where people can pursue their goals without interference. When citizens are empowered to lead their own lives, they contribute to a stronger and more vibrant nation.

The Founding Fathers designed the Constitution to protect against government overreach by establishing checks and balances. Preserving these safeguards ensures that power remains distributed and no branch or institution exceeds its authority. Upholding these principles protects the liberties of every individual, ensuring that government serves the people rather than controlling them.

Championing Individual Liberty:

Why It Matters:

Individual liberty forms the cornerstone of a free society. It means that each person has the fundamental right to determine the course of their life—to set personal goals, nurture their family, and pursue their passions—without excessive constraints. When governments impose unnecessary restrictions, these freedoms erode, and citizens risk losing the ability to shape their destinies. By championing individual liberty, we protect the space where personal responsibility, innovation, and moral judgment can thrive.

Respecting individual liberty doesn't mean ignoring the common good; instead, it acknowledges that progress emerges when free people work together, guided by conscience and shared values rather than forced mandates. Balancing order and freedom ensures that while basic rules safeguard public well-being, individuals retain the dignity and autonomy at the heart of the American spirit.

Guided Meditation:

Close your eyes and take three slow, deep breaths. Imagine standing in a wide-open field under a clear sky, limitless in its expanse. Feel a gentle breeze whispering possibilities and self-determination.

As you breathe in, sense the freedom to make choices about your life—your work, beliefs, relationships, and ambitions. Visualize the barriers of overreach and needless mandates dissolving, leaving you free to shape your world responsibly.

Inhale again, feeling gratitude for your trust in acting ethically and thoughtfully. You sense that with liberty comes respecting others' rights, ensuring everyone may flourish.

Before opening your eyes, envision your community thriving in this freedom— neighbors pursuing different paths yet united by a shared respect for one another's autonomy. Carry this vision with you, remembering that when we champion individual liberty, we preserve the fertile ground where hope, opportunity, and integrity grow.

Affirmation:

"I embrace my liberty with gratitude and responsibility, knowing that freedom empowers me to shape my destiny and respect the choices of others."

Journaling Prompts:

Reflect on a time you exercised personal freedom in a way that enriched your life. What did that experience teach you about the value of autonomy?

Consider how respecting each person's liberty might improve understanding and cooperation within your community. How does freedom encourage empathy and innovation?

Imagine a scenario where excessive rules limit creativity and self-determination. What would be lost in that environment, and how might individual liberty help restore balance?

Practices in Action:

Stay Informed: Learn about local and national regulations that affect your daily life. Understanding these measures allows you to advocate for rights that preserve personal freedom.

Engage in Community Dialogue: Discuss individual liberty and government overreach with friends, neighbors, and community groups. Thoughtful, respectful conversation can inspire positive changes that maintain everyone's autonomy.

Conclusion:

Championing individual liberty ensures everyone can chart their course, guided by conscience, reason, and personal values. When we resist unnecessary interference, we nurture a society where free individuals cooperate voluntarily, honor one another's dignity, and foster a vibrant, enduring spirit of independence. In this balance, we find the space for genuine progress and shared prosperity.

Respecting State & Local Authority:

Why It Matters:

The principle of decentralized power is fundamental to America's democratic framework. It acknowledges that local communities are best equipped to understand and address the needs of their residents. By respecting state and local authority, we ensure that decision-making remains close to the people it impacts, fostering solutions tailored to each community's unique values, challenges, and priorities. When given the autonomy to act, local governments can respond more swiftly and effectively to the needs of their citizens, creating environments where residents feel seen and heard.

State and local governments are better positioned to experiment with innovative policies that reflect their citizens' desires without being burdened by a distant, one-size-fits-all mandate. This decentralized approach strengthens democracy by empowering communities to solve problems that align with their specific needs and values. Respecting this balance of power not only preserves local autonomy but also strengthens national unity, as it reinforces the idea that America's diversity can be its greatest strength.

Guided Meditation:

Close your eyes and take three deep, grounding breaths. Imagine standing in the heart of a small town, where every building, street, and gathering space reflects the unique values of its people. The city is vibrant and alive with activity, and everyone is actively contributing to the well-being of their community.

Picture yourself walking down the main street, passing neighbors collaborating on projects that address their local concerns—cleaning parks, creating new opportunities for small businesses, or hosting town hall meetings to discuss important issues. You feel a sense of pride in these solutions that reflect their distinct needs and culture.

As you breathe in, sense the energy and power from local involvement. These decisions are shaped by people who live, work, and raise their families in this place—who understand it better than anyone else. Exhale, feeling a deep appreciation for the decentralized power that empowers communities to be their architects of change.

Before you open your eyes, imagine this town thriving with innovative policies that benefit everyone—its success is a testament to the local authority's wisdom. Carry this vision with you, understanding that respecting state and local authority allows communities to thrive in ways that honor their distinct identities and values.

Affirmation:

"I honor the importance of state and local authority, recognizing that decentralized power empowers communities to create solutions that reflect their unique values and needs."

Journaling Prompts:

Reflect on a time when local decisions—whether in your town or neighborhood—positively impacted your life. How did this local decision-making improve the community?

Consider how your community's unique needs and values might differ from others. How can state and local governments provide better, more effective solutions when they can act independently?

Envision a future where states and localities have more authority to govern themselves. How might this decentralization lead to more tailored and effective policies?

Practices in Action:

Engage with Local Governance: Attend city council meetings, participate in local forums, or volunteer for community-based organizations. Understanding and engaging with local decisions allows you to advocate for policies that reflect your community's values.

Support Local Solutions: Advocate for policies that allow your local government to have the power to solve issues in the way that best fits your community's needs. Support initiatives that strengthen local decision-making rather than centralizing authority.

Conclusion:

Respecting state and local authority is vital to maintaining a government that is responsive, flexible, and connected to its citizens. By empowering local communities to solve problems that reflect their unique cultures and priorities, we ensure that solutions are practical and deeply rooted in the values that make each community unique. This decentralization strengthens local and national unity, proving that when communities are trusted with the autonomy to make decisions, they flourish in ways that benefit everyone.

Challenging Bureaucratic Expansion:

Why It Matters:

A society weighed down by endless regulations and mandates risks becoming rigid, stagnant, and unresponsive to the people it aims to serve. Over time, excessive bureaucratic expansion can choke innovation, discourage entrepreneurs, and constrain personal freedom. When every decision must pass through layers of red tape, opportunities shrink, and creativity often leads to conformity. Challenging this expansion means advocating for streamlined, sensible governance that prioritizes clarity, efficiency, and the empowerment of individuals.

By resisting unnecessary complexity, we allow fresh ideas to flourish and ensure people have the freedom to pursue their aspirations. This balanced approach doesn't dismiss the role of government—it reaffirms that the government should enable progress, not stand in its way. Embracing fewer, more focused regulations encourages a culture where self-reliance, ingenuity, and personal responsibility guide the path forward.

Guided Meditation:

Close your eyes and take three calming breaths. Imagine walking through a forest of tangled vines representing layers of rules and mandates. The thick undergrowth makes it hard to see a clear way forward, slowing your steps and testing your patience.

As you continue, envision yourself carefully cutting away unnecessary vines, clearing a path that allows light to filter through. The forest becomes less oppressive with each breath, revealing new growth beneath the cleared ground—small saplings of ideas and enterprises waiting to thrive.

Inhale deeply and feel the relief as the path opens. There's no room to move freely, to experiment, to innovate. The weight of excessive regulations fades, replaced by the confidence that people can solve problems and build their futures without needless obstacles.

Before opening your eyes, picture a vibrant clearing where neighbors, entrepreneurs, and creators share ideas. You stand among them, grateful for the space that allows everyone's potential to unfold. Carry this vision forward as a reminder that we nurture opportunity and liberty by challenging bureaucratic expansion.

Affirmation:

"I value streamlined, sensible governance, trusting that fewer unnecessary regulations foster innovation, opportunity, and personal freedom."

Journaling Prompts:

Think of a time when excessive rules or processes hindered your ability to accomplish a goal. How did it affect your motivation and creativity?

Consider how reducing unnecessary mandates could influence entrepreneurship in your community. What new ventures might emerge if people faced fewer bureaucratic barriers?

Envision a future where regulations only support fairness, safety, and essential services. How would this environment encourage individuals to realize their dreams and contribute to society?

Practices in Action:

Stay Informed and speak up: Learn about local and national regulations that affect your personal or professional life. Contact representatives or engage in public forums to advocate for more efficient, balanced policies.

Support Reform Efforts: Support initiatives that simplify and clarify rules for small businesses, nonprofits, and community projects. Doing so, you help create an atmosphere that stimulates growth rather than stifles it.

Conclusion:

Challenging bureaucratic expansion isn't about discarding all rules but freeing individuals, communities, and businesses from needless constraints. In doing so, we ensure that bright ideas and personal ambitions have room to breathe and flourish. Ultimately, trimming unnecessary regulation opens the way to a society defined by innovation, opportunity, and the liberty to forge our paths forward.

Promoting Transparency & Accountability:

Why It Matters:

A healthy democracy depends on trust—trust that those in positions of authority will act honestly, ethically, and in the public's best interest. When elected officials operate in the shadows or cater to special interests above the people they represent, this trust erodes the foundation of our governance. Promoting transparency and accountability means ensuring leaders answer for their actions, explain their decisions, and place citizens' needs front and center.

Exposing governmental processes discourages corruption and empowers citizens to hold their representatives accountable. This clear-eyed approach ensures that policies are based on principles and practical benefits rather than political favors or hidden agendas. In an environment of honesty and responsibility, citizens are more engaged, confident, and willing to participate, knowing their voices truly matter.

Guided Meditation:

Close your eyes and take three steady breaths. Imagine standing in a bright, open hall filled with sunlight. This hall represents the channels of government—every door, window, and walkway is visible, allowing you to see how decisions are made.

As you walk through this space, notice officials engaged in conversation. They speak openly about their intentions, proposals, and the rationale behind their votes. Information flows freely, and nothing important is hidden in dark corners.

Feel a sense of relief and empowerment with every breath. This transparency means leaders know their actions are seen and evaluated by the public. They are accountable, encouraging honesty and ensuring policies serve everyone—not just a privileged few.

Before opening your eyes, imagine citizens calmly asking questions and leaders respectfully responding. Carry this vision forward as a reminder that when we demand openness, we elevate the governance standards and restore trust in the institutions that shape our lives.

Affirmation:

"I stand for transparency and accountability, insisting that leaders govern honestly and responsibly, always putting the people's interests first."

Journaling Prompts:

Recall a time when clear information about a public policy helped you feel more confident in your government's decisions. How did transparency influence your perspective?

Consider what measures—such as public hearings, accessible records, or independent oversight—can improve accountability among elected officials. How might these tools strengthen trust within your community?

Envision a future where leaders habitually explain their choices, seek public input, and uphold ethical standards. How would this impact civic engagement and the quality of life in your area?

Practices in Action:

Stay Informed and ask Questions: Monitor local and national policies, attend public forums or town halls, and politely press representatives for clarification when details seem unclear or incomplete.

Support Reforms That Encourage Openness: Advocate for laws, regulations, or community initiatives that make government records more accessible, increase campaign funding disclosure or establish watchdog groups that monitor officials' conduct.

Conclusion:

Promoting transparency and accountability ensures that the government operates under the watchful eyes of the people it serves. By demanding honesty from elected officials, we create a political culture that rejects secrecy and cronyism. This approach fosters genuine trust, energizing citizens to participate more fully in the democratic process and guiding the nation closer to the ideals upon which it was founded.

Encouraging Self-Reliance & Responsibility:

Why It Matters:

Self-reliance and personal responsibility have long been hallmarks of the American spirit, fueling innovation, entrepreneurship, and resilience. When individuals and families take the lead in managing their lives—rather than relying heavily on distant agencies—they gain confidence, hone problem-solving skills, and strengthen their communities from the ground up. This approach acknowledges that people know their circumstances best and that personal initiative often sparks more meaningful and enduring solutions than top-down directives.

Encouraging self-reliance doesn't mean abandoning those in need. It means creating an environment where assistance is a hand-up, not a permanent crutch. We nurture a healthier balance between community support and personal initiative by empowering individuals and families to define their paths. The result is a society where people take pride in their achievements, celebrate progress, and inspire others to embrace the freedom and responsibility woven into American life's fabric.

Guided Meditation:

Close your eyes and take three steady breaths. Picture yourself in a sunny field, wide and open. This field represents the vast array of opportunities before you—paths you might take, goals you might set, and projects you might pursue.

As you walk through this field, notice you carry a small toolkit—your strengths, talents, and experiences. You have what you need to build, create, and adapt. With each breath, feel the quiet confidence that you can trust your abilities.

Imagine envisioning a project that matters—perhaps starting a small business, learning a new skill, or improving your family's well-being. Inhale and sense your determination growing stronger. Exhale and release any fears or doubts that you must wait for someone else's approval or resources.

Before opening your eyes, picture yourself taking the first step toward your goal. You are the driving force behind your journey, supported by a culture that respects personal effort. Carry this feeling forward, knowing that embracing self-reliance enriches your life and inspires others to do the same.

Affirmation:

"I trust in my ability to shape my future, embracing self-reliance and responsibility as the keys to personal and family success."

Journaling Prompts:

Reflect on a challenge you faced and overcame through your determination. What did this experience teach you about your capabilities?

Consider an area where you rely on outside help. Could you gradually assume more responsibility, and how might doing so help you grow?

Envision a community where most people actively seek opportunities to improve their circumstances. How does this mindset affect local businesses, schools, and neighborhoods?

Practices in Action:

Set Personal Goals: Identify a short-term goal that relies primarily on your initiative—learning a new skill, managing your budget, or organizing a community activity. Achieving it reinforces your confidence in your abilities.

Mentor & Share Knowledge: Offer guidance or mentorship to someone in your circle—helping them troubleshoot a problem, learn a skill, or gain independence. By empowering others, you help spread the culture of self-reliance.

Conclusion:

Encouraging self-reliance and responsibility fosters an environment where individuals and families feel empowered to face life's challenges head-on. Freed from excessive dependency on distant agencies, they become architects of their success stories. In supporting a culture of personal initiative and resilience, we ensure that the American tradition of self-determination remains vibrant and accessible to all.

Safeguarding the Constitution's Limits on Power:

Why It Matters:

The Constitution was carefully crafted to prevent any single branch of government from consolidating too much power. The Founders recognized that the strength of a democracy depends on the balance of power between the legislative, executive, and judicial branches. This system of checks and balances ensures that no institution or individual can overreach, safeguarding the freedoms and rights of citizens. By upholding these limits, we protect the integrity of the system designed to serve the people, not dominate them.

In a society where power is distributed and regulated, tyranny becomes less likely, and citizens can trust that their rights are not subject to the whims of one branch or leader. Safeguarding these limits means standing firm against any attempts to centralize control and ensuring that the principles of democracy continue to function as intended. By doing so, we honor the Founders' vision and ensure that their blueprint for a free and just society endures.

Guided Meditation:

Close your eyes and take three slow, deep breaths. Visualize standing in front of a sturdy, balanced structure—perhaps a courthouse or the columns of a government building. This structure represents the Constitution and its carefully designed system of checks and balances.

As you walk around the building, notice its strong foundations and intricate design. Each section—legislative, executive, and judicial—functions independently but relies on the others to maintain stability. Feel the peace that comes from knowing that no single part of the structure is overpowering the others.

With each breath, imagine the air growing clearer and lighter. The integrity of the system is maintained because each part holds its limits. This balance fosters a safe and just environment for all, where no power is unchecked, and the rights of citizens remain protected.

Before opening your eyes, envision this building standing firm and steady for generations, with citizens and leaders alike respecting the boundaries set by the Founders. Carry this vision with you, knowing that safeguarding the Constitution's limits ensures the enduring strength of freedom.

Affirmation:

"I honor the checks and balances embedded in the Constitution, understanding that these limits protect our freedoms and maintain the balance of power."

Journaling Prompts:

Reflect on the role of the Constitution in shaping the relationship between citizens and government. How does the system of checks and balances ensure fairness and justice?

Consider when you felt that government overreach threatened your freedoms. How can upholding the Constitution's limits prevent such overreach in the future?

Envision a scenario where the balance of power is disrupted. How would this impact the freedoms and rights we take for granted today?

Practices in Action:

Learn & Advocate: Stay informed about the constitutional limits on government power and speak up when you see any branch overstepping its bounds. Support organizations that promote constitutional rights and hold the government accountable.

Engage in Civic Action: Participate in local or national discussions about the importance of the Constitution's checks and balances. Advocate for policies and laws reinforcing these limits and ensuring power remains balanced and distributed.

Conclusion:

Safeguarding the Constitution's limits on power ensures that America remains a nation of liberty, where no single entity can dominate or infringe upon the rights of its citizens. By upholding the Founders' vision of checks and balances, we protect the freedoms that make America unique. In doing so, we maintain a government that is accountable, fair, and focused on serving the people rather than consolidating power.

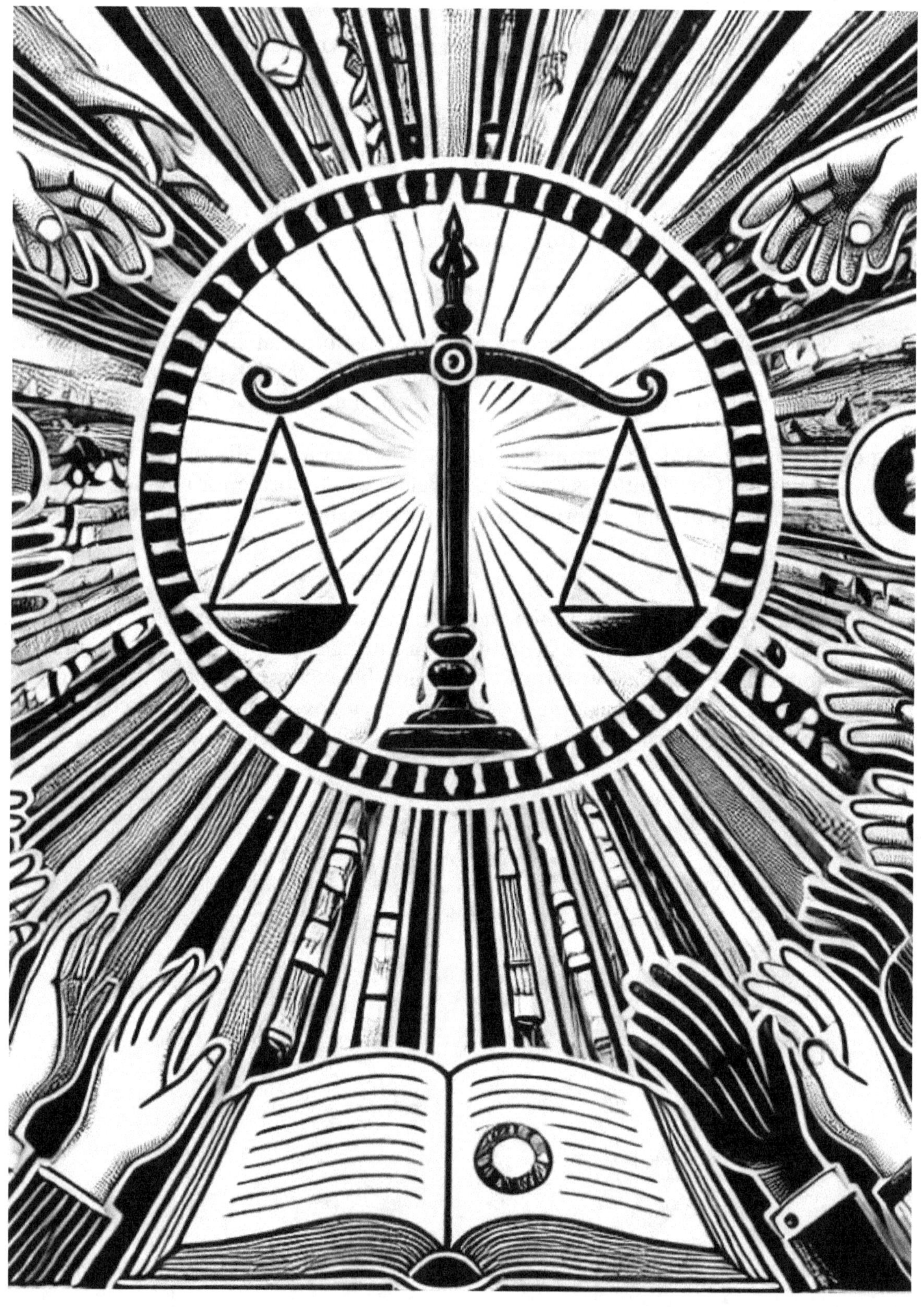

SEVEN: Election Integrity

Free and fair elections are the foundation of any democracy, ensuring that every citizen's voice is heard and that government remains accountable to the people. Election integrity is not a partisan issue—it is a principle that transcends politics and speaks to the heart of a nation's trust in its institutions. Advocacy for stricter voting laws, voter ID requirements, and transparency in the electoral process reflects a commitment to safeguarding democracy and fostering confidence in election outcomes.

The cornerstone of election integrity is a fair and secure system. Stricter voting laws and voter ID requirements help ensure that every ballot cast is valid and represents the will of an eligible voter. These measures protect the integrity of the electoral process, reducing the risk of fraud or abuse while ensuring that every vote is counted accurately.

Transparency is essential for building public confidence in elections. Clear procedures, accessible information, and thorough investigations into alleged irregularities ensure citizens trust the results. Promoting transparency requires openness in elections and accountability when issues arise, reinforcing the legitimacy of democratic processes.

Election integrity involves striking a balance between accessibility and security. While ensuring that every eligible voter has the opportunity to participate is vital, maintaining the integrity of the process is equally important. Measures like secure voting systems, early voting options, and voter education programs can enhance accessibility without compromising security.

Decentralized election management is a hallmark of the American system, allowing states and localities to oversee their processes. Empowering local election officials ensures that systems reflect their communities' unique needs and values while fostering accountability and trust at the grassroots level.

A strong democracy relies on active participation. Encouraging citizens to register, vote, and stay informed about their rights and responsibilities strengthens the electoral process. Civic engagement promotes a culture of involvement and ensures that elections are truly representative of the people.

Election integrity also means ensuring that every eligible voter has fair and equal access to the ballot box. Efforts to make voting accessible—such as clear voter ID guidelines, accessible polling places, and robust voter education—uphold the principle that participation is a right for all citizens.

Ultimately, election integrity is about reinforcing faith in democracy. A secure, transparent, and accessible system fosters unity and trust, encouraging citizens to engage with the process and believe in the outcomes. By advocating for election integrity, we ensure that democracy remains strong and vibrant and reflects people's will.

Ensuring Fair and Secure Elections:

Why It Matters:

The integrity of elections is foundational to the health of any democracy. Ensuring fair and secure polls guarantees that every eligible vote counts while safeguarding the process from fraud, interference, or manipulation. Voter ID requirements, secure voting systems, and transparent procedures help protect the outcome's legitimacy, reinforcing citizens' trust in the democratic process. By ensuring that only eligible voters can cast ballots and that votes are counted accurately, we preserve the fairness and transparency that make elections meaningful.

Advocating for these measures doesn't undermine access to voting but strengthens confidence in the electoral system. When people trust that their votes will be fairly counted, they are more likely to participate, strengthening the foundation of democracy. Ensuring election security benefits everyone, regardless of political affiliation, as it keeps the process equitable and reliable for all.

Guided Meditation:

Close your eyes and take three deep, calming breaths. Imagine standing in a quiet room filled with voters casting their ballots. There's a sense of calm and order here, as each person's voice is heard through their vote.

Picture a simple yet secure voting booth where everyone proudly presents their ID, knowing their vote is crucial and protected. You feel the reassurance of knowing that this system ensures only those eligible participate, strengthening the fairness of the process.

As you inhale, feel the peace that comes with a secure system, knowing that each vote is counted accurately and that no one can tamper with the results. Exhale, releasing any doubts or worries about election integrity. The system is working as it should, and every vote matters.

Before opening your eyes, imagine a community where citizens feel confident in the election system. This trust builds a stronger, more engaged society. Carry this vision forward, knowing that fair and secure elections are key to sustaining democracy.

Affirmation:

"I support secure, transparent elections where every eligible vote counts, fostering trust and confidence in the democratic process."

Journaling Prompts:

Reflect on your personal experience with voting. How does knowing that elections are fair and secure impact your voting decision?

Consider how voter ID requirements and secure voting systems can help prevent fraud while ensuring all eligible voters can access the polls. How do these measures build confidence in the system?

Envision a future where election integrity is beyond question. How might this strengthen democracy and encourage citizens to engage in the electoral process?

Practices in Action:

Educate Yourself and Others: Learn the steps to ensure election security in your area and share this information with others. Knowledge breeds trust.

Encourage Civic Participation: Advocate for transparent election practices and encourage others to vote and engage with the process. Promote the importance of secure elections to safeguard democracy for future generations.

Conclusion:

Ensuring fair and secure elections upholds the very essence of democracy. By advocating for measures that protect the integrity of the electoral process—like voter ID requirements and secure voting systems—we foster a system where every vote counts and every citizen has confidence in the outcome. In doing so, we maintain the trust that is essential for a functioning democracy, one where all people are empowered to shape their future through their votes.

Empowering Local Election Oversight:

Why It Matters:

State and local control over election processes is a cornerstone of American democracy. Empowering local election oversight ensures that communities' unique needs, values, and concerns are reflected in elections. When elections are managed at the state and local levels, residents have greater access to officials who understand their specific circumstances and are more accountable to the people they serve.

Decentralized election oversight also builds trust. It allows communities to set up systems tailored to their population size, geography, and resources rather than relying on one-size-fits-all mandates from distant authorities. This approach ensures greater transparency and fosters confidence in the integrity of the voting process, strengthening the bond between citizens and their electoral system.

Guided Meditation:

Close your eyes and take three slow, calming breaths. Picture yourself standing in your local polling place on Election Day. You see familiar faces—neighbors, community leaders, and volunteers—working together to ensure the voting process runs smoothly.

Imagine walking through the polling area and seeing the care and precision with which ballots are handled and counted. Each detail reflects your community's unique needs and values, managed by people who live and work among you. Feel the sense of trust and accountability this local oversight creates.

Inhale deeply, feeling proud that your community actively ensures fair and accessible elections. Exhale any doubts about the process, knowing that local control prioritizes transparency and responsiveness.

Before opening your eyes, envision the results being tallied with care, overseen by local officials committed to upholding their trust. Carry this vision forward, appreciating the importance of local election oversight in preserving democracy.

Affirmation:

"I value the role of state and local election oversight, trusting that community-led processes ensure fair, transparent, and accountable elections."

Journaling Prompts:

Reflect on how local election oversight fosters trust in the voting process. How does knowing your community manages its elections build confidence in the system?

Consider your area's unique needs, such as population size or geography. How does state or local control allow election systems to serve these needs better?

Envision an election in your community managed entirely by local officials. What steps could be taken to improve accessibility, transparency, or efficiency?

Practices in Action:

Engage Locally: Volunteer as a community poll worker or election monitor. By contributing to the process, you gain firsthand insight into the importance of local control.

Advocate for Decentralization: Support policies that protect state and local authority over election processes. Discuss with neighbors how community-driven oversight benefits voters and strengthens democracy.

Conclusion:

Empowering local election oversight ensures that elections are conducted to reflect the values and needs of the people they serve. By keeping election management close to home, we build trust, enhance accountability, and preserve the integrity of the democratic process. In honoring this principle, we affirm that elections are not just about ballots but about empowering communities to shape their future with confidence and clarity.

Promoting Confidence in Election Outcomes:

Why It Matters:

Trust in the democratic process is essential for a healthy and functioning democracy. When voters feel confident that their ballots are counted accurately and fairly, they are more likely to participate and engage in shaping the future of their communities and the nation. Promoting confidence in election outcomes involves ensuring transparency in the vote-counting process, promptly addressing concerns, and conducting thorough investigations into irregularities.

Transparency and accountability provide a clear public record that builds trust and counters misinformation. By addressing questions or doubts openly and honestly, we create an electoral process that citizens can believe in, regardless of the outcome. Fostering this trust strengthens democracy and ensures that elections serve as a unifying force, bringing communities together through shared civic participation.

Guided Meditation:

Close your eyes and take three slow, steady breaths. Picture yourself standing in a large, well-lit room where votes are being counted. Observers from all sides watch quietly, ensuring the process is transparent and fair.

Imagine the calm, methodical work being done by election officials—each ballot carefully handled, each vote accounted for. See the transparency in their actions and the dedication to accuracy that protects the integrity of the process.

With each breath, feel the sense of security from knowing the system is designed to address concerns openly. Every doubt is met with a clear and honest answer, and irregularities are investigated with precision and care.

Before opening your eyes, visualize a community gathering after the election results are announced. Regardless of differing opinions, people trust the process, knowing their voices are heard. Carry this vision forward, understanding that confidence in election outcomes unites citizens.

Affirmation:

"I trust in the integrity of fair, transparent elections, knowing that openness and accountability build confidence in democratic outcomes."

Journaling Prompts:

Reflect on a time when you felt confident in the results of an election. What factors contributed to your trust in the process?

Consider how transparency in vote counting and addressing irregularities can prevent division and foster unity. How might these practices improve future elections?

Envision an election where every citizen feels their vote was accurately counted regardless of the outcome. What steps can communities take to promote this level of trust?

Practices in Action:

Support Transparency Efforts: Advocate for policies that ensure public access to election oversight, such as live-streaming vote counts or publishing detailed results reports. Transparency builds confidence.

Engage in Election Observation: Volunteer as a poll observer or election monitor to witness the process firsthand and help promote trust in your community.

Conclusion:

Promoting confidence in election outcomes strengthens the foundation of democracy. We create a process that voters can trust by emphasizing transparency, addressing irregularities, and ensuring accurate vote counting. This trust encourages greater participation and helps elections serve their ultimate purpose: giving every citizen a voice in the decisions that shape our future.

Protecting Against Fraud and Abuse:

Why It Matters:

The right to vote is one of the most fundamental freedoms in a democracy, and safeguarding that right requires vigilance against vulnerabilities in the electoral system. Protecting against fraud and abuse ensures that only eligible citizens can cast ballots and are counted accurately. By addressing these vulnerabilities, we maintain the integrity of elections and reinforce public confidence in their outcomes.

Preventing tampering or interference isn't just about preserving the technical aspects of voting—it's about honoring the voices of every voter and ensuring they are heard. A secure electoral process encourages participation, deters terrible actors, and strengthens the bond of trust between citizens and their government. When elections are protected against fraud and abuse, we preserve the foundation of democracy itself.

Guided Meditation:

Close your eyes and take three deep breaths. Picture yourself standing at the threshold of a secure voting center. Inside, you see calm, orderly processes in motion, with officials carefully verifying voter identities and ensuring every step is transparent and fair.

Imagine casting your vote and knowing it is securely recorded. Each voter around you is doing the same, and their ballots are protected from interference or fraud. Inhale deeply, feeling the confidence that comes from knowing the system is designed to uphold the integrity of every vote.

As you exhale, visualize layers of safeguards—advanced technology, vigilant election workers, and independent observers—working together to protect against vulnerabilities. Each measure strengthens your trust in the process and affirms the sanctity of the election.

Before opening your eyes, picture a future where every voter participates in a process free from tampering or abuse, regardless of their background or beliefs. Carry this vision forward, knowing that secure elections are the bedrock of a thriving democracy.

Affirmation:

"I support measures that protect elections from fraud and abuse, ensuring that every vote is cast and counted with integrity."

Journaling Prompts:

Reflect on why preventing fraud and abuse in elections is essential. How does this effort strengthen your trust in democracy?

Consider what steps can be taken to address vulnerabilities in the electoral process without creating unnecessary barriers for eligible voters. How can these efforts balance security and accessibility?

Imagine an election system that all citizens universally trust. What policies or safeguards might be necessary to achieve this?

Practices in Action:

Educate Yourself & Advocate for Security: Learn how elections are secured in your area and advocate for additional measures where needed. Encourage policies that balance accessibility with robust protections against fraud.

Participate in Safeguarding Elections: Volunteer as a poll worker, monitor, or advocate for election reforms. Your involvement helps create a more secure and trustworthy process.

Conclusion:

Protecting against fraud and abuse ensures that elections remain fair, secure, and reflective of the people's will. By addressing vulnerabilities and implementing safeguards, we honor voters' trust in the democratic process. By preserving the integrity of every vote, we reinforce the strength and legitimacy of our democracy, inspiring confidence in current and future generations.

Encouraging Civic Engagement:

Why It Matters:

Civic engagement is the heartbeat of democracy, actively empowering citizens to shape their future. Encouraging participation in elections—through voter registration, casting ballots, and staying informed—ensures that every voice is heard and every perspective is represented. When citizens understand their voting rights and responsibilities, they are better equipped to make decisions that reflect their values and aspirations.

Promoting civic engagement strengthens communities and reinforces the connection between individuals and their government. Voting isn't just an act—it's a declaration of hope and a commitment to progress. By fostering a culture of participation, we ensure that democracy thrives, that leaders remain accountable, and that future generations inherit a system built on active, informed citizenry.

Guided Meditation:

Close your eyes and take three deep breaths. Picture yourself standing in a bustling community center on Election Day. Around you, people of all ages and backgrounds cast their votes, united in the shared act of shaping the future.

Imagine the energy in the room—a sense of pride and determination as each person steps forward to make their voice heard. Feel the connection between these individuals, each contributing to the democratic process uniquely.

With each breath, visualize this participation spreading beyond the voting booth— neighbors registering voters, families discussing issues, and friends encouraging one another to stay informed. Sense the ripple effect of engagement as it strengthens your community's bonds of trust and collaboration.

Before opening your eyes, picture a nation where civic engagement is celebrated and embraced, where every citizen understands the power of their vote. Carry this vision forward, knowing that participation is the foundation of a thriving democracy.

Affirmation:

"I embrace my role as an engaged citizen, knowing that by voting and staying informed, I help shape a brighter future for all."

Journaling Prompts:

Reflect on your own voting experiences. What emotions or thoughts come to mind when you participate in elections?

Consider what motivates people to vote or stay informed. How can these motivations be strengthened to encourage broader civic engagement?

Envision ways you could inspire others—family, friends, or neighbors—to participate in the democratic process. What impact might this have on your community?

Practices in Action:

Help Others Register to Vote: Volunteer with organizations that assist with voter registration, ensuring that as many citizens as possible are ready to participate in upcoming elections.

Promote Awareness: Share information about voting rights, deadlines, and responsibilities with your community. Encouraging others to stay informed helps build a culture of engagement.

Conclusion:

Encouraging civic engagement ensures that democracy remains vibrant and inclusive. When citizens participate—by registering, voting, and staying informed—they shape the policies and leaders that guide their lives. This active involvement creates a more representative government and strengthens the bonds that hold our communities together. By fostering participation, we safeguard the principles of democracy and ensure a brighter future for all.

Safeguarding Equal Access to Voting:

Why It Matters:

Voting is a cornerstone of democracy, and ensuring equal access to the ballot box is essential for a system that represents all voices. Balancing security measures with accessibility helps maintain the integrity of elections while ensuring that no eligible voter is left out. By making voting both secure and straightforward, we uphold the principle that every citizen's voice deserves to be heard.

Efforts to safeguard equal access to voting involve addressing barriers that might deter participation, such as long wait times, limited polling locations, or overly complex requirements. At the same time, these efforts include implementing measures that protect the process from fraud or tampering. Striking this balance ensures elections remain fair, inclusive, and reflective of the diverse perspectives within the nation.

Guided Meditation:

Close your eyes and take three slow, steady breaths. Imagine a smooth, well-lit path leading to a polling station. Along the way, you see people of all ages and backgrounds walking confidently toward the same destination, knowing their right to vote is respected and protected.

Picture the polling station as a welcoming space—organized, efficient, and accessible. There are no barriers here, just an open invitation for every eligible voter to cast their ballot securely and efficiently. Feel the sense of unity and empowerment from this shared civic participation act.

With each breath, envision the harmony of a process that balances security and accessibility. You see safeguards in place to protect the integrity of the vote, but these measures never hinder anyone's ability to participate. Each vote carries equal weight and is counted with care.

Before opening your eyes, imagine a nation where voting is both a right and a celebration. Every citizen feels confident that the system is fair, inclusive, and secure. Carry this vision with you, knowing that safeguarding equal access strengthens democracy for all.

Affirmation:

"I believe in balancing election security with accessibility, ensuring that every eligible voter has an equal opportunity to vote confidently and easily."

Journaling Prompts:

Reflect on the importance of equal access to voting. How does ensuring fairness and inclusivity strengthen your trust in the democratic process?

Consider challenges that might prevent eligible voters from participating in elections. What solutions could address these issues while maintaining election security?

Envision an election process where no voter feels excluded or discouraged. What steps could your community or nation take to realize this vision?

Practices in Action:

Support Accessibility Initiatives: Advocate for measures that make voting easier for all, such as extended voting hours, mail-in ballots, and accessible polling locations.

Help Others Participate: Encourage neighbors, family members, or friends to register to vote, find their polling place, or understand their voting rights. Your encouragement can make a significant difference.

Conclusion:

Safeguarding equal access to voting ensures that democracy remains inclusive and representative of all voices. By balancing security with accessibility, we uphold the principle that every eligible citizen deserves a fair chance to participate in shaping their future. This commitment to fairness strengthens trust in the electoral process and reinforces the ideals of equality and opportunity that define our nation.

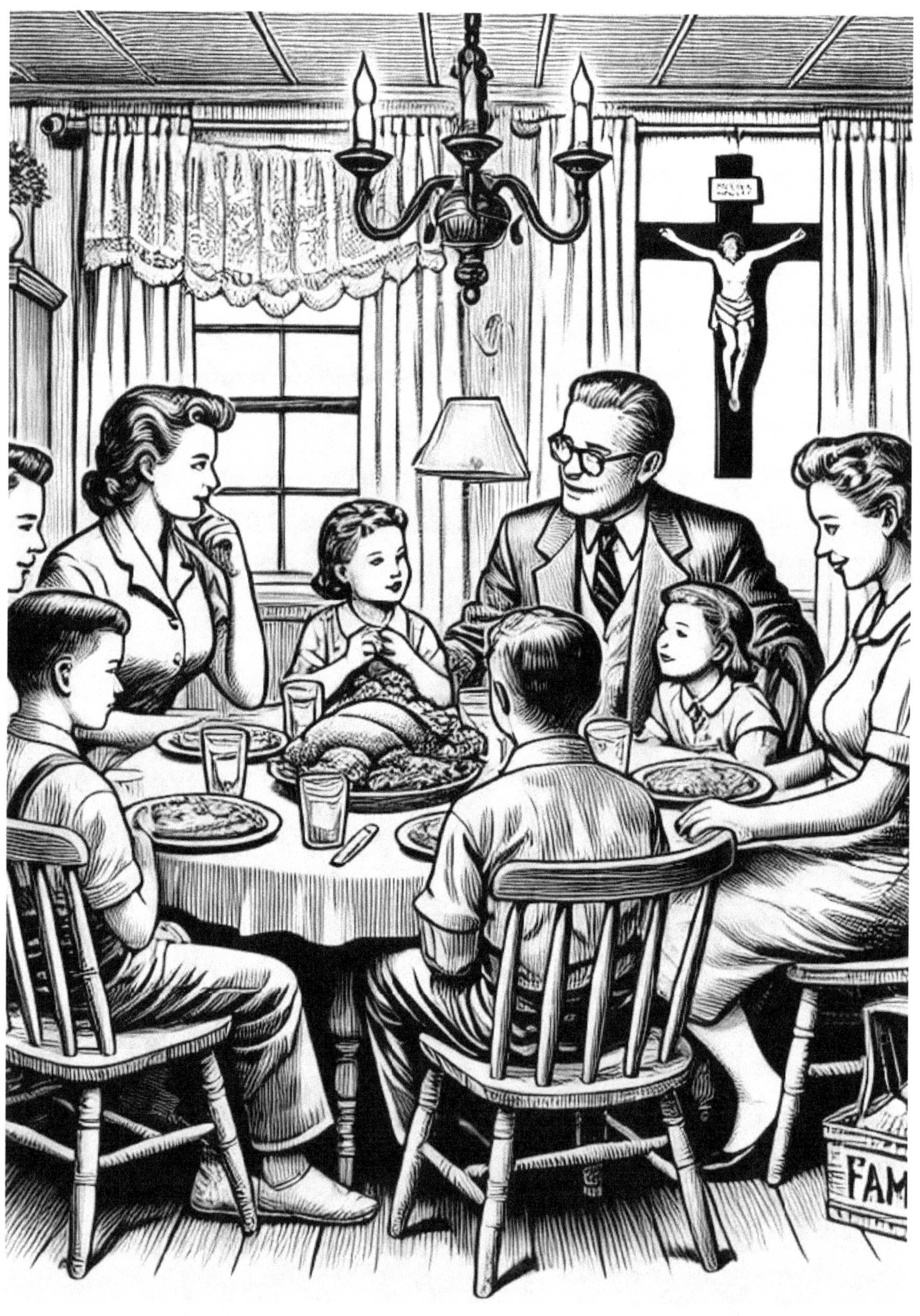

FAM

EIGHT: Traditional Family Values

The family is often called the cornerstone of society, where love, support, and shared values create the foundation for personal and communal growth. Traditional family values emphasize stable marriages, engaged parenting, and education that reflects the moral and cultural principles families cherish. These values foster environments where individuals can thrive and strengthen relationships and communities flourish.

Stable, loving families provide children the structure to grow into confident, compassionate adults. Policies that strengthen the family unit—through economic assistance, marriage enrichment programs, or parental resources—help create homes where love, respect, and responsibility are taught and practiced. A strong family is the bedrock of a strong society.

Traditional family values emphasize the importance of relationships across generations. Grandparents, parents, and children share a legacy of wisdom, stories, and traditions that bind them together. Honoring these intergenerational bonds nurtures respect and connection, ensuring that moral values and cultural heritage are preserved for future generations.

Education plays a critical role in passing down family values. Schools emphasizing respect, responsibility, and empathy reinforce the lessons taught at home, preparing children to navigate life with integrity and understanding. Advocating for values-based education ensures curricula align with the principles families hold dear while fostering environments where character development is prioritized.

Parenting is one of the most important responsibilities a person can undertake. Traditional family values celebrate the role of parents as primary guides in their children's moral and emotional development. Supporting responsible parenthood means empowering families with resources, education, and community support to raise children who embody respect, resilience, and kindness.

Faith traditions and community groups are vital in reinforcing traditional family values. These networks provide families spiritual guidance, practical resources, and emotional support, creating a sense of belonging and shared purpose. Encouraging participation in these institutions helps families stay grounded and connected, offering a framework for living out their values in daily life.

Parents are the first and most important teachers in a child's life. Traditional family values prioritize the rights of parents to guide their children's education and upbringing according to their beliefs and principles. Ensuring parents retain this authority strengthens families and fosters a culture of trust, respect, and shared responsibility.

Traditional family values extend beyond individual households, creating stronger neighborhoods and communities. When families thrive, so do schools, workplaces, and local economies. Supporting these values means investing in families at every level, from policy to community programs, ensuring they remain the heart of a healthy, vibrant society.

Strengthening the Family Unit:

Why It Matters:

Strong families are the cornerstone of a thriving society. Stable, loving marriages and close-knit family units provide the foundation for emotional well-being, personal development, and community growth. When families are healthy and supportive, they nurture individuals who contribute positively to society, instilling values like respect, responsibility, and compassion.

Strengthening the family unit isn't just about upholding traditions—it's about recognizing that the bonds of love and trust within families create the building blocks for success and resilience. By promoting policies and practices that support families, we invest in a future where individuals can flourish, communities can grow more substantial, and the ideals of a harmonious and flourishing society can be realized.

Guided Meditation:

Close your eyes and take three steady breaths. Picture yourself standing in the warm glow of a family gathering. Around you, laughter fills the air, stories are shared, and love is present in every interaction. This is a space of stability and connection.

Imagine the bonds between each family member—a web of support, trust, and encouragement. These bonds strengthen with each shared moment and the mutual act of care. Breathe deeply, feeling the security and warmth from being surrounded by love and unity.

Visualize this family as a seedbed of positive values and lifelong lessons. As members support one another, they are empowered to grow and thrive. With every breath, sense the ripple effect of these strong bonds extending outward into the wider community.

Before opening your eyes, imagine your family or the families you know contributing to a thriving society—one where love and responsibility flourish. Carry this vision forward, knowing that strengthening the family unit uplifts everyone.

Affirmation:

"I value the strength and love of the family unit, recognizing it as the foundation of personal growth, community well-being, and societal success."

Journaling Prompts:

Reflect on when your family or a close-knit group supported you through a challenge. How did their love and care help you grow?

Consider the role of family values in shaping individuals. What values or lessons from your family do you hope to pass on to future generations?

Envision a society where every family is stable, supportive, and loving. How would this environment influence communities and future generations?

Practices in Action:

Support Family Time: Dedicate time each week to meaningful family activities, whether shared meals, outdoor adventures, or simply sitting down for a heartfelt conversation. Strengthening these bonds nurtures the entire family.

Advocate for Family-Friendly Policies: Support policies that provide family resources, such as parental leave, affordable childcare, and educational opportunities. These measures help create a stable foundation for families to grow and thrive.

Conclusion:

Strengthening the family unit ensures that society is built on a foundation of love, trust, and mutual support. We nurture individuals who carry these positive values into their communities by fostering stable marriages and close-knit family bonds. In prioritizing the well-being of families, we create a society where everyone can flourish and contribute to a brighter, more harmonious future.

Honoring Intergenerational Bonds:

Why It Matters:

Intergenerational bonds are vital threads in the fabric of family life. These connections link generations, allowing grandparents, parents, and children to share wisdom, stories, and traditions. When families celebrate these bonds, they preserve moral values and cultural heritage, grounding younger generations in a sense of identity and purpose. Grandparents offer a perspective shaped by time, passing on lessons that guide and inspire, while grandchildren bring fresh energy and hope, creating a cycle of mutual enrichment.

Honoring these bonds strengthens the family as a unit, fostering more profound respect, understanding, and love among its members. By nurturing connections across generations, families create a legacy of shared values, ensuring that the principles that guide them today continue to flourish in the future.

Guided Meditation:

Close your eyes and take three steady breaths. Picture yourself sitting in a warm, welcoming room where three generations of your family gather. Grandparents share stories, children listen intently, and parents facilitate the connection with pride and love.

Imagine the wisdom these stories share—tales of resilience, faith, and hope. Each word builds a bridge between the past and the future. Breathe deeply, feeling the weight of these lessons settle in your heart as they become part of your story.

Envision how these bonds enrich both young and old. Grandparents find joy in their role as guides and mentors, while children feel empowered by the love and guidance of their elders. Each generation uplifts the others, creating a cycle of growth and renewal.

Before opening your eyes, imagine these bonds extending outward, weaving a tapestry of love, heritage, and shared values that strengthen the family. Carry this vision forward, knowing that honoring intergenerational bonds enriches everyone involved.

Affirmation:

"I celebrate the wisdom and love shared across generations, knowing that strong family ties preserve our values and cultural heritage for the future."

Journaling Prompts:

Reflect on a lesson or tradition from an elder in your family. How has this wisdom influenced your life and values?

Consider how you can nurture relationships with your family's older and younger generations. What actions might strengthen these bonds?

Envision your family as a chain of connected generations. What legacy would you like to pass on to your children, grandchildren, or community members?

Practices in Action:

Spend Time Together: Plan activities that bring multiple generations of your family together, such as sharing a meal, playing games, or discussing family history. These moments build lasting connections.

Preserve Family Stories: Interview elders in your family about their lives, values, and traditions. Document their stories to share with future generations, ensuring their wisdom endures.

Conclusion:

Honoring intergenerational bonds celebrates the richness of family life and the wisdom that flows through it. Families connect younger and older generations to build a bridge between the past and the future, preserving moral values, cultural heritage, and love. In fostering these bonds, we create a legacy that empowers individuals and strengthens the family, enriching today and future generations.

Advocating for Values-Based Education:

Why It Matters:

Education shapes the character and future of individuals and society alike. Advocating for values-based education ensures schools impart knowledge and nurture qualities like respect, responsibility, and empathy. When educational curricula align with the moral and ethical principles taught at home, they reinforce a cohesive foundation for children to grow into compassionate, moral adults.

Values-based education fosters a balanced approach to learning, combining academic excellence with social and emotional development. By emphasizing respect for others, accountability for actions, and understanding diverse perspectives, this approach equips students with the tools they need to succeed personally and professionally. Strengthening the connection between family values and educational principles ensures children grow up with a consistent and supportive framework for navigating the world.

Guided Meditation:

Close your eyes and take three steady breaths. Imagine sitting in a classroom filled with eager, curious students. The walls are adorned with inspiring messages about kindness, integrity, and perseverance. This space is designed to nurture both knowledge and character.

Picture a teacher guiding a lesson on facts and life values—helping students learn about respect, responsibility, and empathy. With each word, the students grow more confident in contributing positively to the world.

Inhale deeply, feeling the warmth of a shared commitment between families and schools to nurture these values. Exhale, releasing doubts about whether children will find their way—they are surrounded by support and guidance.

Before opening your eyes, envision these students taking their lessons into the world, carrying the values cherished at home and reinforced in school. Carry this vision forward, confident that values-based education creates a brighter future for all.

Affirmation:

"I advocate for education that nurtures respect, responsibility, and empathy, aligning with the values cherished at home to guide children toward lives of purpose and integrity."

Journaling Prompts:

Reflect on when you saw values like respect or empathy demonstrated in an educational setting. How did it impact the students involved?

Consider the values most important to you and your family. How could schools better incorporate these principles into their curricula?

Envision a classroom where respect, responsibility, and empathy are as central to learning as math or reading. What outcomes would you expect for students and their communities?

Practices in Action:

Engage with Schools: Attend school board meetings or parent-teacher conferences to advocate for educational programs emphasizing character development and academics.

Model Values: Volunteer at local schools or mentor students, demonstrating the importance of respect, responsibility, and empathy through your actions.

Conclusion:

Advocating for values-based education bridges the gap between home and school, creating a cohesive environment where children can thrive. Integrating respect, responsibility, and empathy into curricula prepares students to succeed academically and grow into compassionate, moral individuals. In fostering this alignment between family values and education, we build a society where character and knowledge go hand in hand, ensuring a future guided by shared ideals.

Promoting Responsible Parenthood:

Why It Matters:

Parents are a child's first and most influential teachers, shaping their moral compass, emotional resilience, and understanding of the world. Promoting responsible parenthood emphasizes the importance of parents as active participants in their children's development, nurturing values like respect, empathy, and integrity. By providing love, guidance, and stability, parents lay the foundation for their children's success and the future strength of society.

Recognizing the vital role of parents doesn't mean expecting perfection—it's about encouraging intentional and compassionate parenting. When parents take responsibility for their children's growth, they instill a sense of accountability for future generations. Supporting parents in this role ensures that families remain the cornerstone of a thriving and values-driven society.

Guided Meditation:

Close your eyes and take three deep breaths. Picture yourself in a peaceful home surrounded by the laughter and energy of children. The air is filled with warmth and love, and you feel responsible for guiding these young lives.

Imagine sitting with a child, listening attentively to their questions, fears, and dreams. You feel more connected with every breath, knowing that your words and actions leave a lasting imprint on your heart and mind.

Envision moments of teaching—showing them the importance of kindness, patience, and honesty. Picture the joy in their eyes as they learn these lessons, carrying them into their future relationships and endeavors.

Before opening your eyes, picture this child growing into an adult who embodies your instilled values. Carry this vision with you, knowing that your role as a parent is a profound and sacred contribution to the world.

Affirmation:

"I embrace the role of a responsible parent, nurturing my children's moral and emotional growth and shaping their future with love, guidance, and integrity."

Journaling Prompts:

Reflect on a value or lesson you learned from your parents or guardians. How has this influenced the way you approach parenting or guiding others?

Consider the qualities of responsible parenthood—patience, consistency, empathy—and how they impact children's development. Which of these qualities do you strive to embody?

Envision a society where every parent feels supported as a guide and mentor. What changes might emerge in families and communities?

Practices in Action:

Prioritize Quality Time: Dedicate daily time to connect with your children, whether through shared activities, meaningful conversations, or simply listening to their thoughts and feelings.

Seek Support & Resources: Take advantage of parenting classes, community resources, or mentorship opportunities to strengthen your parenting skills and confidence.

Conclusion:

Promoting responsible parenthood acknowledges parents' profound influence on their children's lives. By serving as loving guides, parents instill values, build emotional resilience, and shape the character of future generations. Supporting and celebrating the role of parents ensures that families remain strong, communities thrive, and society benefits from the foundation of love and responsibility.

Encouraging Faith & Community Support:

Why It Matters:

Faith traditions, community groups, and local mentors are invaluable in nurturing spiritual growth and reinforcing healthy values within families and individuals. These networks provide support, guidance, and encouragement, offering a sense of belonging and shared purpose. Faith and community-based initiatives often serve as pillars of strength during difficult times, helping individuals navigate challenges with resilience and hope.

By fostering connections between families and these supportive networks, we ensure that no one faces life's challenges alone. These institutions promote compassion, integrity, and accountability while cultivating a spirit of service to others. Encouraging faith and community support uplifts individuals and strengthens the bonds that create thriving, values-driven societies.

Guided Meditation:

Close your eyes and take three deep, steady breaths. Imagine yourself standing in the heart of a welcoming community space—a church, a local center, or a neighbor's gathering. This place radiates warmth and unity, a haven where everyone is valued.

Picture the people around you sharing stories, offering encouragement, and helping one another. As you breathe deeply, feel the strength of being part of a group that shares your values and works together to uplift everyone.

Envision the lessons learned in this space—kindness, humility, and caring for others. Let these teachings flow into your heart, inspiring you to carry them daily.

Before opening your eyes, imagine this community expanding, welcoming more people, and nurturing future generations. Carry this vision with you, knowing that faith and community support provide a foundation for personal and collective growth.

Affirmation:

"I celebrate the role of faith traditions and community support in nurturing values, fostering resilience, and strengthening the bonds that unite us."

Journaling Prompts:

Reflect on a time when faith, a community group, or a mentor provided you with guidance or encouragement. How did this experience shape your values or strengthen your resolve?

Consider how community involvement or participation in faith traditions can positively impact families and individuals. What role do these networks play in your life or your community?

Envision a society where everyone can access a supportive network of faith and community groups. How would this transform relationships and the well-being of families?

Practices in Action:

Engage with Community Groups: Participate in local faith traditions, volunteer organizations, or mentorship programs. Building connections through these networks fosters a sense of belonging and shared purpose.

Offer Support: Be a mentor or active participant in your community, helping others navigate challenges and find strength through shared values and encouragement.

Conclusion:

Encouraging faith and community support highlights the importance of connection, shared values, and mutual care. By embracing these networks, individuals and families find the strength and guidance to grow spiritually and morally. Together, these institutions create a society grounded in compassion, resilience, and service, ensuring that every person feels supported and empowered to lead a life of purpose and fulfillment.

Prioritizing Parental Rights in Education & Upbringing:

Why It Matters:

Parents are uniquely equipped to understand their children's needs, values, and aspirations. Prioritizing parental rights in education and upbringing ensures that decisions about how children learn, grow, and thrive remain in those who know them best. While schools and policymakers play a role in shaping educational systems, parents must retain the authority to guide their children's development in ways that align with their family's values and priorities.

This principle reinforces the importance of family autonomy in determining what is best for each child. By ensuring parents have a say in education and upbringing, we foster environments where children are supported holistically—academically, morally, and emotionally. Empowering parents this way nurtures confident, well-rounded individuals and strengthens the bond between families and communities.

Guided Meditation:

Close your eyes and take three deep breaths. Picture yourself sitting at a kitchen table with your child, discussing their dreams and interests. You feel a deep sense of responsibility and pride in guiding them on their unique path.

Imagine actively shaping your child's education, selecting the books they read, the subjects they study, and the values they learn. Each decision you make is thoughtful and will reflect your family's principles and your child's potential.

Inhale deeply, feeling the confidence that comes with knowing you are the primary influence in your child's growth. Exhale, releasing any concerns about distant policymakers dictating their future. The power to guide your child's upbringing rests where it belongs—in your hands.

Before opening your eyes, envision your child thriving, their education and upbringing reflecting the love and care you've poured into them. Carry this vision forward, trusting parental rights' importance in shaping their journey.

Affirmation:

"I honor the role of parents as the primary guides in their children's education and upbringing, ensuring every decision reflects their love, values, and aspirations."

Journaling Prompts:

Reflect on your parents or guardians' influence on your upbringing and education. How did their guidance shape who you are today?

Consider the balance between parental authority and external educational policies. What steps can be taken to ensure parents have the most significant say in their children's learning and development?

Envision an educational system where parents actively shape curricula and policies. How would this improve child outcomes and strengthen families?

Practices in Action:

Get Involved in Education: Attend school board meetings, engage with teachers, and participate in parent-teacher organizations to ensure your voice is heard in your child's educational journey.

Advocate for Parental Rights: Support policies and initiatives that empower parents to have a more significant say in their children's education and upbringing, fostering systems that reflect family values.

Conclusion:

Prioritizing parental rights in education and upbringing ensures children grow up with guidance rooted in love, understanding, and shared values. When parents are empowered to influence their children's development, they create environments where learning and growth are tailored to their needs. By affirming the authority of families over distant policymakers, we strengthen the bonds of trust and responsibility that lead to healthier, happier, and more successful generations.

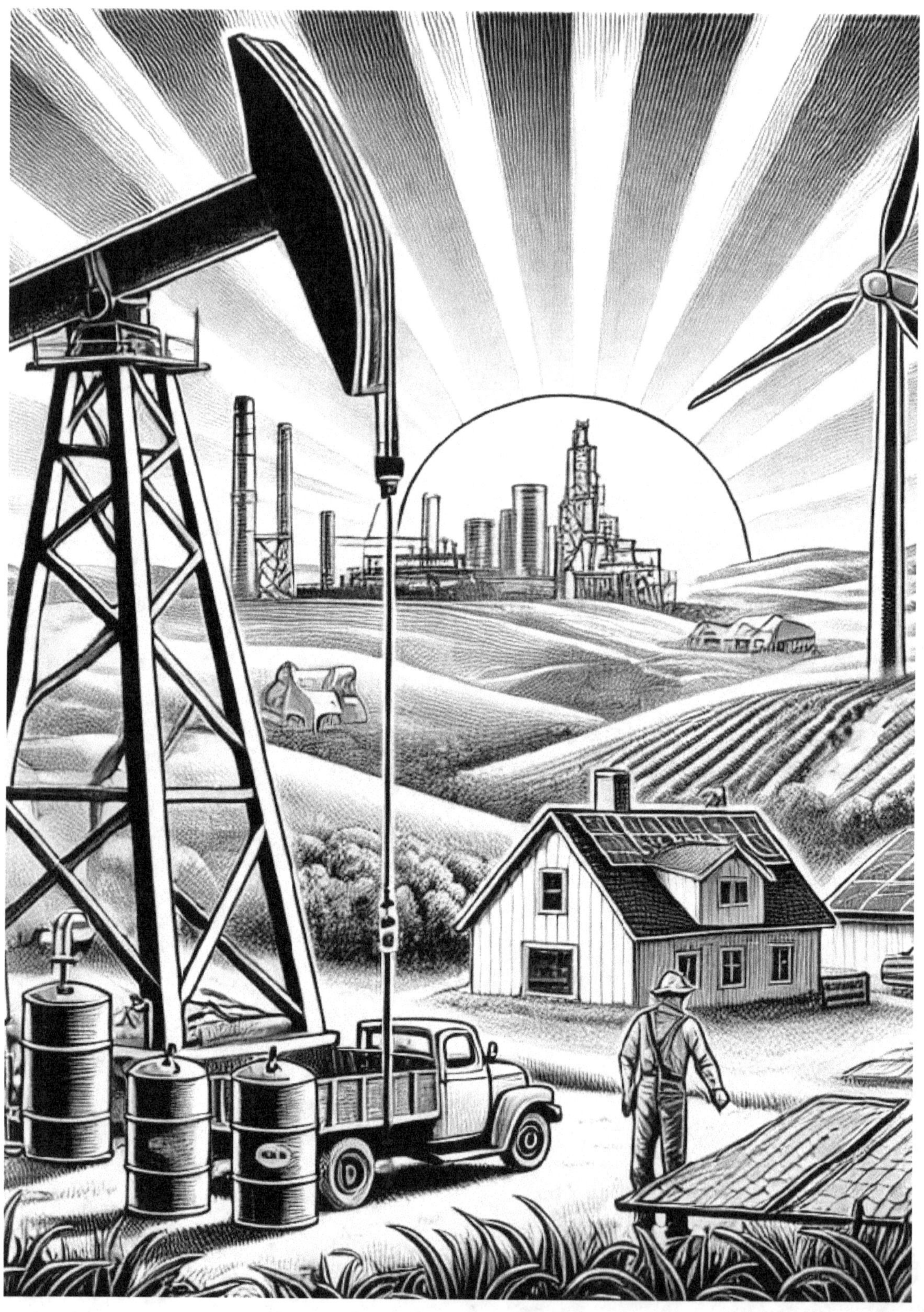

NINE: Energy Independence

Energy independence is essential for a secure and prosperous nation. By prioritizing domestic energy production—including oil, natural gas, and coal—the United States reduces its reliance on foreign suppliers, ensuring stability and self-reliance in an unpredictable global market. Energy independence protects national security, fuels economic growth, supports local communities, and creates jobs that strengthen the American workforce.

America is rich in natural resources, and tapping into these reserves responsibly strengthens the economy while providing reliable energy for homes, businesses, and critical infrastructure. Revitalizing domestic industries such as oil, natural gas, and coal fosters job creation, innovation, and economic self-reliance. It ensures that energy needs are met without overreliance on external sources, securing a more stable future.

Dependence on foreign energy sources leaves the nation vulnerable to supply disruptions and price fluctuations caused by global conflicts or geopolitical tensions. Domestic energy production safeguards national security by ensuring the country has access to the resources it needs to function effectively. A self-reliant energy policy reinforces the ability to protect American interests at home and abroad.

Energy independence stabilizes prices, providing predictable costs for families and businesses. Sudden spikes in energy prices can strain household budgets and disrupt economic growth. By producing energy domestically, the U.S. ensures a steady supply that supports affordability and prevents market volatility, allowing communities to plan for the future confidently.

While oil, natural gas, and coal play a vital role in current energy needs, investing in research and innovation lays the foundation for a more sustainable future. Cleaner extraction methods and advancements in alternative energy sources such as wind, solar, and advanced batteries enhance efficiency while reducing environmental impact. A commitment to innovation ensures that America remains a global energy production and technology leader.

Energy independence does not mean sacrificing the environment. Responsible development includes adopting practices that minimize environmental impact, protect ecosystems, and promote sustainability. By balancing energy growth with environmental care, we demonstrate that economic progress and preservation can go hand in hand, benefiting current and future generations alike.

Energy independence also involves empowering states and local communities to harness their natural resources. Tailored approaches that reflect local values and needs ensure that energy development benefits the people most directly affected. This localized approach strengthens economies, supports communities, and reinforces the connection between citizens and the resources that power their lives.

Revitalizing Domestic Industries:

Why It Matters:

Energy independence is more than a policy goal—it's a pathway to economic growth, national security, and innovation. By revitalizing domestic industries such as oil, natural gas, and coal, the U.S. reduces reliance on foreign energy sources while creating jobs and supporting local economies. Tapping into homegrown energy resources provides stability and security, shielding the country from global market fluctuations and ensuring that energy needs are met reliably and affordably.

Revitalizing these industries also fosters innovation, encouraging advancements in cleaner, more efficient energy technologies. When energy production thrives at home, communities benefit from strengthened economies, new opportunities, and a renewed pride in their contributions to national progress. Supporting domestic energy development ensures a brighter, more secure future for all.

Guided Meditation:

Close your eyes and take three deep breaths. Picture a bustling energy production site in the heart of America. Workers are active, machinery hums steadily, and the air is filled with determination and purpose.

Imagine the positive ripple effects of this industry—jobs created, local businesses thriving, and families supported. Breathe deeply, feeling the pride and confidence from knowing your community contributes to the nation's energy needs.

Envision innovation emerging from these efforts. As domestic industries expand and adapt, cleaner technologies, more innovative solutions, and more efficient processes arise. With each breath, sense the balance of progress and preservation, securing economic growth and environmental stewardship.

Before opening your eyes, picture a strong, self-reliant America powered by its resources and ingenuity. Carry this vision forward, knowing that revitalizing domestic industries strengthens the economy and the nation.

Affirmation:

"I support revitalizing domestic energy industries, recognizing their role in creating jobs, fostering innovation, and ensuring America's energy independence."

Journaling Prompts:

Reflect on how energy production impacts your local or national economy. What benefits have you seen or could you imagine from revitalizing domestic industries?

Consider the relationship between energy independence and national security. How does reducing reliance on foreign energy sources strengthen the country's position?

Envision a future where domestic energy industries lead the world in innovation and sustainability. What steps can be taken to achieve this balance?

Practices in Action:

Support Local Energy Initiatives: Learn about and advocate for domestic energy projects in your community, including oil, natural gas, coal production, and cleaner energy technologies.

Encourage Innovation: Back efforts to develop advanced energy solutions that make domestic industries more efficient and sustainable, ensuring long-term growth and resilience.

Conclusion:

Revitalizing domestic industries is a cornerstone of energy independence, creating economic opportunities while strengthening national security. By tapping into America's resources and fostering innovation, we secure a future where communities thrive, families benefit, and the nation remains strong and self-reliant. In embracing these efforts, we power a brighter, more sustainable tomorrow for future generations.

Strengthening National Security:

Why It Matters:

Energy independence is closely tied to national security. By producing and utilizing our energy resources—such as oil, natural gas, and coal—the United States reduces its reliance on foreign suppliers, many of whom may have conflicting interests or unstable markets. Strengthening self-reliance in energy ensures that critical infrastructure, military operations, and everyday needs are not vulnerable to disruptions caused by global conflicts or geopolitical tensions.

Domestic energy production enhances stability and control over the nation's energy future, insulating the country from price fluctuations and supply chain vulnerabilities. A firm, self-sufficient energy policy safeguards national interests and provides a foundation for economic and military resilience, reinforcing the security and well-being of all Americans.

Guided Meditation:

Close your eyes and take three deep breaths. Picture a map of the United States, its vast resources glowing like veins of light beneath the surface. These resources represent the energy reserves that power homes, industries, and national defense.

Imagine the country utilizing these resources efficiently and responsibly, reducing reliance on distant, unpredictable suppliers. With each breath, feel the steady strength that comes from knowing America's energy needs are met from within, secure from external disruptions.

Envision how this independence fortifies national security. Military operations have reliable energy sources, critical infrastructure operates without interruption, and families rest easier knowing that energy availability is not subject to foreign instability.

Before opening your eyes, picture an America that stands strong and self-reliant, its energy security bolstering its economy and global position. Carry this vision forward, knowing that producing our energy resources enhances the safety and stability of the nation.

Affirmation:

"I support domestic energy production, knowing it strengthens America's self-reliance, stability, and national security."

Journaling Prompts:

Reflect on how energy independence contributes to national security. Why is reducing reliance on foreign suppliers critical for protecting American interests?

Consider the vulnerabilities that come from dependence on foreign energy. How might domestic production shield the nation from disruptions or conflicts?

Envision a future where America's energy needs are fully met through domestic resources. How would this enhance stability and security for future generations?

Practices in Action:

Stay Informed About Energy Policy: Learn about policies and initiatives prioritizing domestic energy production and consider supporting measures that enhance national security through self-reliance.

Advocate for Resilient Infrastructure: Encourage investment in energy infrastructure that supports economic growth and military readiness, ensuring secure access to resources.

Conclusion:

Strengthening national security through energy independence ensures that America remains self-reliant and protected from external threats. By prioritizing domestic production, we safeguard critical systems, enhance stability, and reduce vulnerability to geopolitical risks. In supporting these efforts, we build a nation that is stronger, safer, and better prepared to face the challenges of the future.

Protecting Affordability & Stability:

Why It Matters:

Energy is a fundamental part of daily life, powering homes, businesses, and infrastructure. Protecting energy affordability and stability ensures that families heat their homes, businesses operate effectively, and communities thrive without sudden cost spikes or supply shortages. When energy prices remain stable and predictable, families can plan their budgets, and businesses can grow confidently.

A reliable energy supply strengthens the economy and promotes resilience. By prioritizing domestic energy production and streamlining delivery systems, we reduce vulnerability to global market fluctuations or disruptions. Protecting affordability and stability supports individual households and reinforces national economic health, fostering growth and security for all.

Guided Meditation:

Close your eyes and take three deep breaths. Picture your home as warm and well-lit, powered by reliable energy. You feel secure, knowing your family's needs are met without worrying about sudden price increases or power outages.

Imagine your community bustling with activity. Businesses are thriving, schools are running smoothly, and neighbors are confident in their ability to plan for the future. Each breath you take reinforces the stability and peace that come from affordable, reliable energy.

Envision an efficient, sustainable, and secure energy production and distribution network. With every breath, sense the balance of supply and demand, ensuring that families and businesses have consistent access to the energy they need.

Before opening your eyes, picture a nation where energy is accessible, affordable, and stable, providing the foundation for prosperity and resilience. Carry this vision forward, confident in protecting energy affordability and stability.

Affirmation:

"I support efforts to protect affordable and stable energy, ensuring families and businesses can thrive without fear of sudden cost spikes or shortages."

Journaling Prompts:

Reflect on the role stable energy prices play in your daily life. How does affordability impact your ability to plan for the future?

Consider how disruptions in energy supply or rising costs could affect families, businesses, or entire communities. What steps can be taken to minimize these risks?

Envision a future where energy is consistently affordable and accessible for everyone. What policies or innovations might help achieve this stability?

Practices in Action:

Advocate for Energy Stability: Support policies and initiatives that prioritize domestic energy production and improve infrastructure to ensure a reliable and affordable supply.

Educate Others: Share information about the importance of energy stability with your community, encouraging conversations about balancing affordability, sustainability, and growth.

Conclusion:
Protecting affordability and stability in energy ensures that families, businesses, and communities can thrive without unpredictable costs or shortages. We create a foundation for economic resilience and personal security by prioritizing reliable domestic production and effective distribution. Supporting these efforts helps ensure a brighter, more stable future, empowering individuals and businesses to plan and prosper confidently.

Investing in Future Technologies:

Why It Matters:

Investing in future energy technologies is essential for balancing the immediate benefits of domestic energy production with long-term sustainability and environmental stewardship. By encouraging research into cleaner, more efficient extraction methods, the U.S. can use its energy resources responsibly while reducing environmental impact. Simultaneously, exploring alternative and renewable energy sources—like solar, wind, and advanced battery technologies—ensures that the nation remains a leader in innovation and energy independence.

Developing these technologies domestically creates jobs, fosters economic growth, and enhances global competitiveness. By committing to innovation, we position the U.S. as a pioneer in energy solutions, preparing for a future where clean, efficient, and sustainable energy is accessible to all. This dual focus on responsible resource use and renewable energy secures economic and environmental well-being for future generations.

Guided Meditation:

Close your eyes and take three deep breaths. Picture a laboratory with scientists, engineers, and innovators working together to develop cutting-edge energy technologies. The air buzzes with creativity and determination.

Imagine these advancements taking shape—cleaner extraction methods for natural resources, efficient renewable energy systems, and powerful new tools for storage and distribution. Each breath you take reflects the balance of progress and sustainability.

Visualize these innovations being implemented across the country. Communities are powered by clean energy, and industries thrive on new, efficient technologies. Feel the pride of knowing these advancements were developed by American ingenuity.

Before opening your eyes, envision a future where the U.S. leads the world in energy innovation, securing economic strength and environmental health. Carry this vision forward, confident that investing in future technologies benefits people and the planet.

Affirmation:

"I support investment in innovative energy technologies, balancing responsible resource use with sustainable, renewable solutions for the future."

Journaling Prompts:

Reflect on how cleaner extraction methods or renewable energy sources could benefit your community. What positive changes might you see?

Consider the importance of innovation in maintaining energy independence. How can investing in research strengthen both the economy and the environment?

Envision a future with widely used renewable energy sources and responsibly managed traditional energy resources. What steps are necessary to make this vision a reality?

Practices in Action:

Support Renewable Energy Research: Advocate for funding and policies that promote the development of renewable energy technologies and cleaner extraction methods.

Educate Yourself and Others: Learn about emerging energy technologies and share this knowledge with your community, encouraging awareness and discussion about sustainable energy solutions.

Conclusion:

Investing in future energy technologies ensures that America remains at the forefront of innovation while balancing energy independence with environmental responsibility. By fostering cleaner extraction methods and supporting the development of renewable resources, we secure a more sustainable and prosperous future. Embracing this dual focus empowers the U.S. to lead by example, proving that economic growth and environmental care can go hand in hand.

Promoting Environmental Stewardship at Home:

Why It Matters:

Promoting environmental stewardship at home ensures that economic growth and resource development are conducted responsibly, preserving the nation's natural beauty and ecosystems for future generations. Responsible development recognizes that energy production and environmental care can coexist, fostering a balanced approach that respects economic and ecological needs.

This stewardship benefits local communities by protecting air, water, and land quality while supporting industries that rely on sustainable practices. By prioritizing the careful management of resources, we demonstrate a commitment to leaving the environment better than we found it, creating a legacy of prosperity and preservation that strengthens the bond between people and the land they call home.

Guided Meditation:

Close your eyes and take three deep breaths. Picture yourself standing in a vibrant natural landscape—a forest, a coastline, or a rolling plain. The air is fresh, and the environment is alive with thriving plants and wildlife.

Imagine how this balance is maintained through thoughtful, responsible development. Nearby, you see workers and industries operating carefully, ensuring that their activities protect the surrounding environment while contributing to economic growth.

Inhale deeply, feeling the harmony of progress and preservation. Exhale, releasing tension about choosing between growth and environmental care—both are possible through mindful stewardship.

Before opening your eyes, visualize this balance spreading across the nation, where every community thrives alongside well-managed natural resources. Carry this vision forward, knowing that promoting environmental stewardship creates a healthier, more sustainable future.

Affirmation:

"I support responsible development that balances economic growth with carefully managing our nation's resources and ecosystems."

Journaling Prompts:

Reflect on the natural beauty in your local area or favorite places in the U.S. How can responsible development protect these spaces while supporting economic needs?

Consider the balance between economic growth and environmental stewardship. How can individuals, businesses, or governments achieve this harmony?

Envision a future where natural ecosystems and resource development coexist sustainably. What role might you play in fostering this balance?

Practices in Action:

Support Sustainable Practices: Advocate for policies encouraging industries to adopt environmentally responsible methods, ensuring growth and preservation.

Engage Locally: Volunteer with or support community initiatives focused on conservation, tree planting, cleanups, or other activities that protect and enhance local ecosystems.

Conclusion:

Promoting environmental stewardship at home ensures that economic progress does not come at the expense of natural resources or ecosystems. By embracing responsible development practices, we demonstrate that growth and preservation can work hand in hand. This balanced approach safeguards the environment for future generations and creates stronger, healthier communities where prosperity and sustainability go together.

Empowering Local Communities:

Why It Matters:

Empowering local communities to manage their natural resources responsibly fosters solutions that are both effective and reflective of local needs and values. Each state and region has unique resources, challenges, and priorities, and allowing them to tailor resource development ensures that policies align with their communities' specific economic, environmental, and cultural contexts.

When local governments and citizens are given the authority to harness their resources, they create opportunities for economic growth, job creation, and innovation that directly benefit their communities. This localized approach also encourages accountability and sustainable practices, ensuring that development respects the environment and the people who depend on it. Empowering local communities strengthens the bond between individuals and the land they care for, promoting progress grounded in shared responsibility and mutual benefit.

Guided Meditation:

Close your eyes and take three deep breaths. Picture your community—a place where people work together to care for the land, water, and resources they rely on. Shared responsibility fosters both growth and preservation.

Imagine local leaders, families, and businesses collaborating to create resource management plans that reflect the community's values. Each decision is made with care, balancing economic opportunity with environmental stewardship.

Inhale deeply, feeling the pride and connection from seeing your community take charge of its future. Exhale, releasing doubts about whether progress can be achieved responsibly—it can and begins at the local level.

Before opening your eyes, envision a thriving region where tailored solutions meet local needs, creating harmony between resource development and community well-being. Carry this vision forward, knowing that empowering local communities leads to sustainable progress.

Affirmation:

"I support empowering local communities to responsibly harness their natural resources, creating solutions that reflect their unique needs, values, and priorities."

Journaling Prompts:

Reflect on the natural resources in your state or region. How could local management of these resources benefit your community economically and environmentally?

Consider how empowering local communities might create more sustainable and innovative solutions. What examples can you think of where local decision-making has led to positive outcomes?

Envision a future where communities take the lead in resource development. How might this approach strengthen the connection between people and the environment?

Practices in Action:

Engage Locally: Support or participate in initiatives encouraging local resource management and sustainability efforts, such as regional energy projects or conservation programs.

Advocate for Decentralization: Promote policies that empower states and regions to make their own decisions about natural resource development, ensuring these choices reflect the needs of their communities.

Conclusion:

Empowering local communities to manage their natural resources responsibly ensures solutions are tailored to each region's unique needs and values. By fostering local accountability and innovation, this approach creates opportunities for economic growth and environmental preservation that benefit everyone. In supporting these efforts, we build a nation where progress and responsibility go hand in hand, strengthening communities and protecting the land they call home.

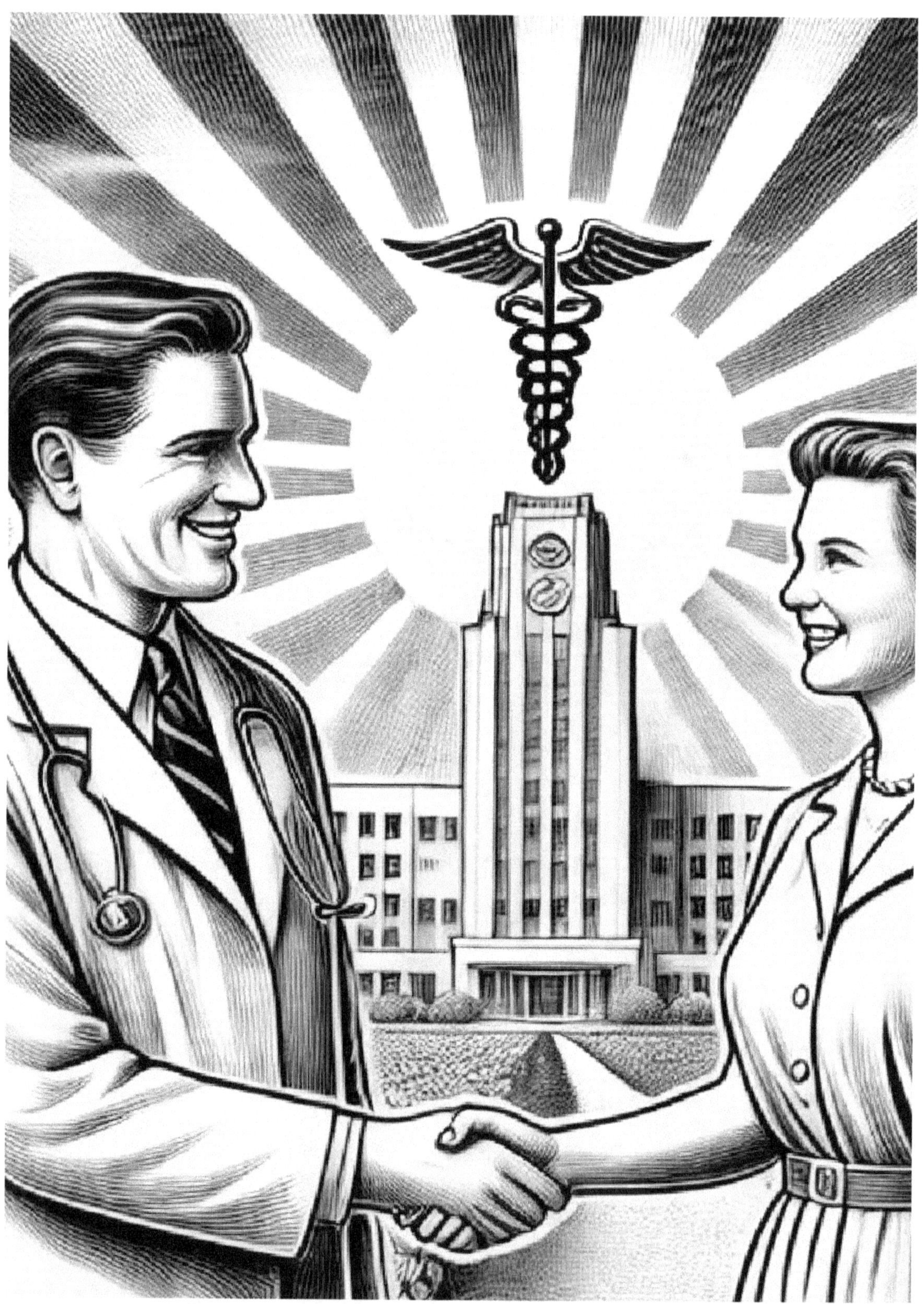

TEN: Healthcare Reform and Freedom

Healthcare is one of life's most personal and impactful aspects, touching every individual, family, and community. Yet, many Americans face rising costs, limited choices, and complex regulations complicating their access to quality care. Healthcare reform is more than improving systems—it's about empowering individuals, lowering costs, and preserving the freedom to make choices that align with personal values and needs.

At the heart of healthcare reform is the principle of autonomy. Individuals should be free to make decisions about their care without being constrained by unwelcome mandates or bureaucratic interference. Whether choosing a doctor, exploring treatment options, or selecting an insurance plan, personal choice ensures that healthcare remains responsive and tailored to individual needs.

High drug prices and rising healthcare costs place significant burdens on families, making life-saving treatments and preventive care unattainable for many. Advocating for transparent pricing, competitive markets, and policy changes that address these challenges ensures that quality care becomes affordable and accessible. Lowering costs doesn't just alleviate financial strain—it improves health outcomes and creates a more equitable system.

Healthcare reform should prioritize patients, focusing on solutions that respect their unique circumstances and values. Shifting away from one-size-fits-all guidelines toward a more personalized approach ensures that individuals feel heard and supported. Care becomes more effective and meaningful when doctors and patients collaborate on treatment plans without interference from distant entities.

Advances in medical research, telehealth, and care delivery systems offer exciting opportunities to make healthcare more efficient and accessible. By encouraging innovation, we can reduce wait times, improve patient satisfaction, and reach underserved communities. Investing in future technologies strengthens the healthcare system and ensures that care adapts to patients' evolving needs.

Trust is the foundation of effective healthcare. Preserving the doctor-patient relationship ensures that decisions are guided by expertise, compassion, and collaboration rather than administrative pressures. Supporting policies that empower doctors to focus on their patients without excessive red tape strengthens this essential bond, improving outcomes for everyone.

Excessive regulations often create unnecessary barriers to care, diverting resources and time away from patients. Simplifying and streamlining these regulations allows healthcare professionals to focus on what matters most: healing and innovation. A flexible, efficient system ensures patients receive the necessary care without delays or unnecessary complications.

Healthcare reform is about creating a system that works for all Americans. By empowering individuals, lowering costs, and fostering innovation, we can ensure that care is accessible, affordable, and responsive. A reformed healthcare system respects personal freedom, supports providers, and prioritizes the well-being of patients, creating a healthier and more compassionate nation.

Empowering Personal Choice:

Why It Matters:

Empowering personal choice in healthcare ensures that individuals can make decisions that best suit their needs, values, and circumstances. Healthcare is deeply personal, and excessive mandates or government interference can undermine people's trust and autonomy to navigate their well-being. By prioritizing personal choice, we affirm that individuals are best equipped to determine their healthcare paths in consultation with trusted medical professionals.

This approach encourages innovation and competition in the healthcare industry, driving better quality, accessibility, and affordability. When individuals have more control over their healthcare decisions, they can seek solutions that align with their financial and personal priorities, creating a system that is both flexible and responsive.

Guided Meditation:

Close your eyes and take three calming breaths. Picture yourself in a quiet, welcoming doctor's office. You feel confident and at ease, knowing you can choose your healthcare path without external pressure or mandates.

Imagine discussing your options with a trusted medical professional and exploring treatments and plans that reflect your values and priorities. Each breath you take reinforces your trust and respect in this partnership.

Visualize yourself, making decisions freely, guided by the best information available and your intuition. With each breath, sense the empowerment from knowing your health choices are entirely your own.

Before opening your eyes, picture a healthcare system where everyone has access to the resources, professionals, and freedom needed to manage their well-being. Carry this vision forward, confident that empowering personal choice creates a healthier, more responsive system for all.

Affirmation:

"I support the right of individuals to make their own healthcare decisions, free from unwelcome mandates and excessive interference."

Journaling Prompts:

Reflect on a healthcare decision you or someone close to you made. How did having the freedom to choose impact the outcome or your sense of control?

Consider the potential challenges of balancing personal choice with ensuring access and affordability. What solutions might address these concerns while maintaining individual autonomy?

Envision a healthcare system where every person feels empowered to make informed decisions about their care. What changes or policies would help achieve this?

Practices in Action:

Stay Informed: Research your healthcare options, from insurance plans to treatment choices, to ensure you make decisions that align with your needs and values.

Advocate for Choice: Support policies that expand access to affordable healthcare options while preserving individuals' right to choose what's best for them.

Conclusion:

Empowering personal choice in healthcare ensures that individuals retain control over decisions directly affecting their lives. We create a more flexible, responsive, compassionate system by prioritizing autonomy and reducing unwelcome interference. In supporting these efforts, we uphold the principle that healthcare is personal and that the best decisions are made by those directly involved in their care.

Reducing Costs & Increasing Access:

Why It Matters:

Affordable and accessible healthcare is essential for a thriving and equitable society. Reducing costs while increasing access ensures everyone can obtain the care they need without facing insurmountable financial burdens. Transparent pricing and competitive markets empower patients to make informed choices, driving down costs and improving the overall quality of care.

High drug prices and unaffordable healthcare often put vital treatments out of reach for many families. By advocating for policy changes that encourage fair competition and price transparency, we create a system where quality care is no longer a privilege but a basic standard. This approach strengthens the connection between healthcare providers and patients, ensuring the focus remains on healing and well-being.

Guided Meditation:

Close your eyes and take three deep breaths. Picture yourself in a pharmacy or doctor's office where the costs of treatments and medications are displayed and easy to understand. You feel relieved knowing you can make informed choices about your care.

Imagine a healthcare system where no one can choose between paying for treatment and meeting other basic needs. See families, individuals, and seniors confidently accessing the care they need without fear of financial strain.

With each breath, visualize a market where innovation flourishes, and competition keeps prices fair. Feel reassured that quality care is available to everyone, regardless of income or circumstances.

Before opening your eyes, picture a future where healthcare is affordable, accessible, and transparent. Carry this vision forward, confident that reducing costs and increasing access strengthens individuals and society.

Affirmation:

"I support efforts to reduce healthcare costs and increase access, ensuring quality care is affordable and available to all who need it."

Journaling Prompts:

Reflect on when healthcare costs impacted your decisions or those of someone you know. How could transparent pricing or lower costs have improved the situation?

Consider how competitive markets and policy changes might lower drug prices and healthcare costs. What specific reforms do you believe would be most effective?

Envision a healthcare system where everyone can access affordable care. How would this change the well-being of families, communities, and society?

Practices in Action:

Educate Yourself on Pricing: Research healthcare providers and pharmacies that offer transparent pricing and lower-cost options. Share this information with friends and family to promote informed choices.

Advocate for Reform: Support policies encouraging competition, reducing costs, and ensuring fair pricing for medications and treatments. Your voice can help drive meaningful change.

Conclusion:

Reducing costs and increasing access to healthcare is a critical step toward creating a system that works for everyone. By promoting transparent pricing and competitive markets, we lower barriers to quality care and ensure no one is left behind. Supporting these efforts fosters a healthier, more equitable society where individuals and families can focus on well-being without the burden of financial strain.

Prioritizing Patient-Centered Solutions:

Why It Matters:

Healthcare is deeply personal, and every patient's needs, values, and circumstances are unique. Prioritizing patient-centered solutions ensures that care is designed around the individual rather than rigid bureaucratic guidelines. This approach respects the humanity of each patient, fostering better outcomes by tailoring treatments, plans, and options to align with their specific situations.

Patient-centered care encourages collaboration between healthcare providers and patients, building trust and empowering individuals to participate actively in their health. By focusing on flexibility and respect, we create a healthcare system that values quality over quantity, promoting well-being through understanding and compassion.

Guided Meditation:

Close your eyes and take three steady breaths. Picture yourself sitting with a compassionate healthcare provider who listens carefully to your concerns, values, and goals. You feel genuinely heard and understood.

Imagine the provider discussing various options tailored to your needs. With each breath, you sense the care and thoughtfulness in their recommendations, reflecting your medical situation and personal preferences.

Visualize yourself as an active partner in your healthcare decisions, fully informed and supported. Inhale deeply, feeling empowered to choose the path that best aligns with your unique circumstances. Exhale any frustration or helplessness, knowing your voice is central to the process.

Before opening your eyes, picture a healthcare system where every patient feels respected and valued, with care designed to honor their individuality. Carry this vision forward, knowing patient-centered solutions build a more compassionate and effective system.

Affirmation:

"I support patient-centered healthcare solutions that respect each individual's unique needs, values, and circumstances."

Journaling Prompts:

Reflect on when a healthcare provider truly listened to your needs or those of someone you care about. How did that experience impact the quality of care?

Consider the benefits of shifting healthcare focus from standardized guidelines to patient-centered solutions. What changes would this bring to the system and patient outcomes?

Envision a future where every healthcare decision prioritizes the individual's voice and circumstances. How might this approach strengthen trust and improve care quality?

Practices in Action:

Advocate for Personalized Care: Encourage friends, family, and community members to seek providers who prioritize patient-centered solutions and share resources about finding compassionate, flexible care.

Engage in Dialogue: When visiting healthcare providers, openly communicate your values and preferences to ensure your care reflects your unique needs.

Conclusion:

Prioritizing patient-centered solutions transforms healthcare into a system that truly serves the individual. By respecting each patient's circumstances, values, and needs, we foster trust, improve outcomes, and create a compassionate environment for healing. Supporting this approach ensures that healthcare focuses on its most important mission: caring for people with dignity and understanding.

Promoting Innovative Care Models:

Why It Matters:

Innovation is the key to addressing many challenges in modern healthcare. Promoting innovative care models—such as medical breakthroughs, telehealth, and advanced delivery systems—can significantly improve efficiency, reduce wait times, and enhance patient satisfaction. These advancements empower healthcare providers to reach more people while offering personalized, high-quality care.

Telehealth, for example, allows patients to consult with providers from the comfort of their homes, making healthcare more accessible to rural communities, busy professionals, and those with mobility challenges. Meanwhile, breakthroughs in treatments and new care models bring hope and solutions to those with complex conditions. By fostering innovation, we build a healthcare system that is more responsive, flexible, and effective, ensuring that patients receive the care they need when and how they need it.

Guided Meditation:

Close your eyes and take three deep breaths. Picture yourself in a world where accessing healthcare is simple, quick, and efficient. You pick up your phone or computer, and within moments, you're connected to a caring provider who listens and addresses your concerns.

Imagine breakthroughs in treatments—innovative therapies and technologies that offer new hope for previously untreatable conditions. With every breath, feel the excitement of living in a time when innovation makes healthcare more effective and accessible.

Visualize the impact of these advancements on patients and providers alike. Waiting rooms are less crowded, care is tailored to individual needs, and satisfaction is high. Inhale deeply, sensing the balance between cutting-edge technology and compassionate care.

Before opening your eyes, picture a future where every patient can access innovative care models prioritizing efficiency, convenience, and quality. Carry this vision forward, knowing that promoting innovation improves lives and strengthens the healthcare system.

Affirmation:

"I support innovative care models that enhance efficiency, reduce wait times, and improve access, ensuring a better healthcare experience for all."

Journaling Prompts:

Reflect on how innovations like telehealth or new treatments have impacted your healthcare experience or that of someone you know. How did they improve access, efficiency, or outcomes?

Consider the barriers that might prevent the widespread adoption of innovative care models. How could these challenges be addressed to make advancements more accessible?

Envision a healthcare system fully embracing innovation. How would new care models transform the patient experience and overall satisfaction?

Practices in Action:

Explore Telehealth Options: Research telehealth providers and services in your area to understand how they can offer convenient and efficient care. Share your experiences with others to promote awareness.

Advocate for Innovation: Support policies and initiatives that fund medical research, encourage technological advancements and expand access to new care delivery models.

Conclusion:

Promoting innovative care models brings healthcare into the future, offering solutions that are more efficient, accessible, and patient-centered. By embracing advancements like telehealth and medical breakthroughs, we improve the quality of care while reducing barriers and wait times. Supporting these innovations ensures that the healthcare system evolves to meet the needs of patients in a way that is both modern and compassionate.

Supporting Doctor-Patient Relationships:

Why It Matters:

The doctor-patient relationship is the foundation of effective healthcare. Preserving this trust and autonomy ensures that medical decisions are guided by a collaborative partnership between doctors and patients rather than by distant entities such as insurers or government agencies. This relationship fosters open communication, personalized care, and mutual respect, allowing patients to feel confident and empowered in their treatment plans.

When doctors are free to focus on their patient's unique needs, and patients can trust their providers to act in their best interests, healthcare outcomes improve. Supporting doctor-patient relationships strengthens the human connection at the heart of medicine, ensuring that care remains compassionate, responsive, and aligned with individual circumstances.

Guided Meditation:

Close your eyes and take three deep breaths. Picture yourself in a calm, welcoming doctor's office. Your doctor is seated across from you, listening intently to your concerns and offering thoughtful advice. You feel safe and respected.

Imagine a collaborative conversation where your doctor explains your options and invites your input. With each breath, feel the trust and confidence growing in this partnership, knowing that your unique needs are central to the discussion.

Visualize your decisions, free from external pressures or mandates. Each choice reflects your values and circumstances, guided by the expertise of a trusted medical professional.

Before opening your eyes, picture a healthcare system where every doctor-patient relationship is supported and valued, fostering a culture of trust and autonomy. Carry this vision forward, knowing this connection is key to meaningful and effective care.

Affirmation:

"I support preserving trust and autonomy in doctor-patient relationships, ensuring healthcare decisions are guided by collaboration and compassion."

Journaling Prompts:

Reflect on when a doctor will listen and collaborate with you. How did this experience impact your confidence in the treatment plan?

Consider the potential consequences of external interference in healthcare decisions. How can supporting doctor-patient relationships mitigate these challenges?

Envision a future where patients feel supported and respected in their medical care. What steps can be taken to strengthen the bond between doctors and patients?

Practices in Action:

Choose Providers Thoughtfully: Seek out healthcare providers who prioritize open communication and collaboration and encourage others to do the same.

Advocate for Autonomy: Support policies and initiatives that empower doctors and patients to guide treatment plans without unnecessary interference from insurers or bureaucracies.

Conclusion:

Supporting doctor-patient relationships ensures that healthcare remains personal, compassionate, and effective. By fostering trust and autonomy in medical decisions, we uphold the dignity of providers and patients, creating a system where care is guided by expertise and understanding rather than external pressures. Strengthening this partnership improves outcomes and reinforces the human connection at the heart of healthcare.

Championing Freedom from Overregulation:

Why It Matters:

Excessive regulations and red tape can stifle medical professional's ability to provide timely and effective care. By championing freedom from overregulation, we create an environment where doctors, nurses, and researchers can focus on what truly matters—healing, innovation, and personalized patient care. Simplifying the regulatory landscape improves efficiency and fosters creativity and progress in medical science.

When administrative tasks and unnecessary rules burden healthcare providers, their time and energy are diverted from patients. By challenging these barriers, we empower professionals to work more effectively, build stronger doctor-patient relationships, and advance medical research. This approach creates a more compassionate, responsive, and innovative healthcare system.

Guided Meditation:

Close your eyes and take three steady breaths. Imagine a bustling hospital or clinic where healthcare providers move freely, unencumbered by unnecessary paperwork or excessive rules. Their focus is solely on their patients.

Picture a doctor spending more time with a patient, carefully listening to their concerns, and crafting a personalized treatment plan. With each breath, sense the freedom and focus this simplified environment provides.

Visualize a researcher working in a state-of-the-art lab, unhindered by bureaucratic delays. Their discoveries bring new hope to patients and families. Breathe deeply, feeling the excitement and potential of an environment where innovation flourishes.

Before opening your eyes, imagine a healthcare system where professionals are empowered to prioritize care and creativity. Carry this vision forward, knowing that reducing overregulation fosters better outcomes for everyone.

Affirmation:

"I support reducing excessive regulations in healthcare, empowering professionals to focus on healing, research, and personalized care."

Journaling Prompts:

Reflect on how overregulation might impact healthcare providers and patients. How could reducing administrative burdens improve care quality and access?

Consider the balance between necessary oversight and excessive regulation. What steps can be taken to streamline processes while maintaining accountability and safety?

Envision a healthcare system free from unnecessary red tape. How would this change how providers interact with patients and approach their work?

Practices in Action:

Advocate for Reform: Support policies that streamline healthcare regulations, reduce paperwork and empower professionals to focus on patient care and innovation.

Engage with Providers: Talk to local healthcare professionals about the challenges they face due to regulations and share their insights with policymakers to advocate for meaningful changes.

Conclusion:

Championing freedom from overregulation empowers healthcare professionals to dedicate their time and energy to what matters most—healing, research, and personalized care. Reducing unnecessary administrative burdens creates a more efficient, compassionate, and innovative system. Supporting this effort ensures patients and providers benefit from a healthcare system focused on excellence and humanity.

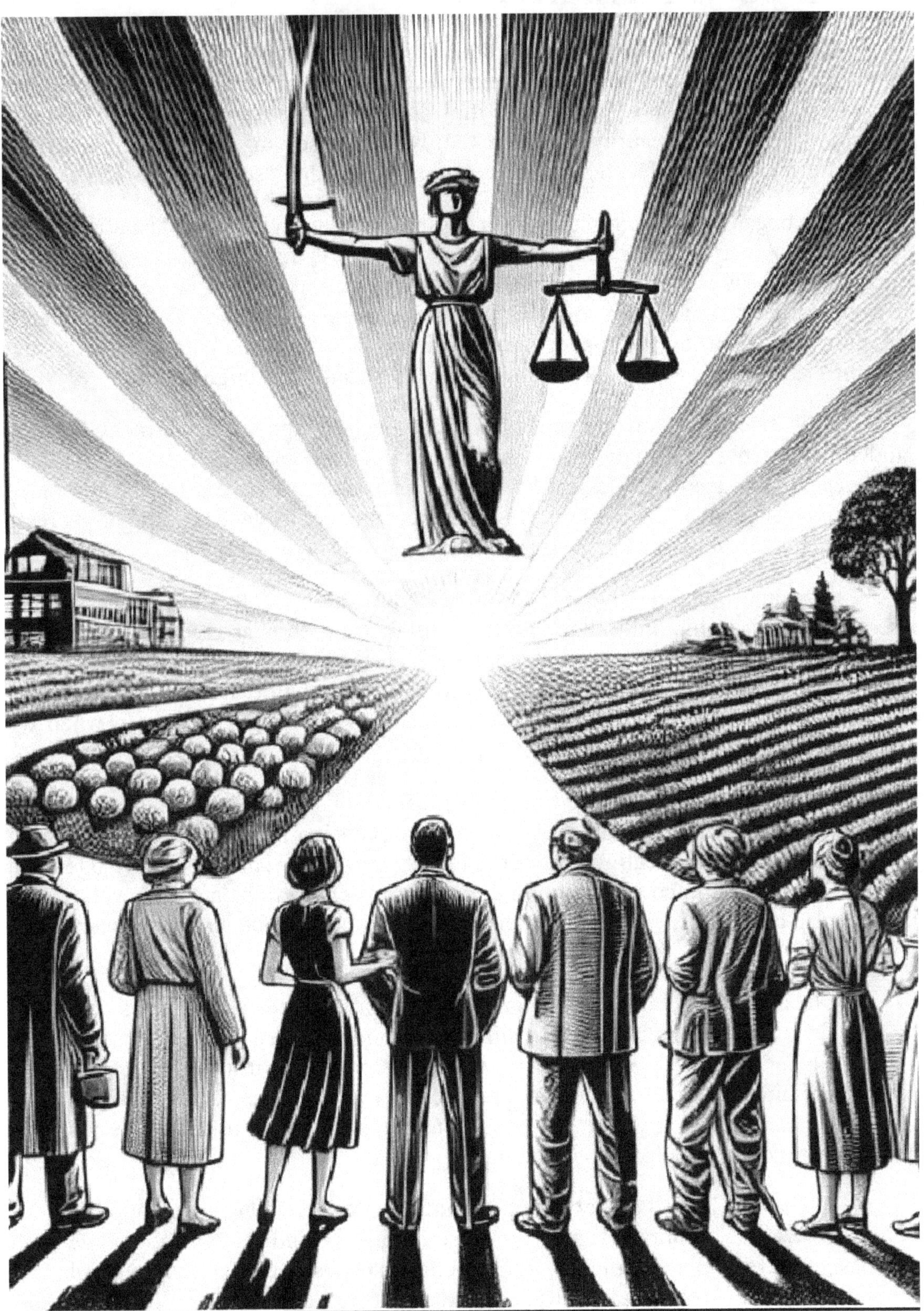

What Have We Learned?

As we conclude this journey through some of the most pressing issues facing our nation, we must reflect on what we have explored and hope to achieve. This book was crafted to illuminate the values and priorities that matter deeply to many Americans—economic opportunity, security, freedom, family, and preserving cherished traditions—while offering thoughtful, actionable ways to engage with these principles daily.

We began by affirming the values defining us as individuals and a nation. From prioritizing American workers and revitalizing local industries to safeguarding Constitutional rights and fostering national sovereignty, this book has celebrated the spirit of resilience, innovation, and unity that drives progress. Each section has explored the unique challenges and opportunities within these domains, emphasizing that positive change begins with understanding and is sustained through action.

This book has encouraged personal reflection and empowerment through guided meditations, affirmations, journaling prompts, and practical steps. These tools were designed to deepen understanding of the issues and inspire clarity and focus. By connecting each reader's values to broader societal concerns, we have sought to create a bridge between individual growth and collective well-being.

In a time when divisiveness can overshadow dialogue, this book has aimed to rise above partisanship and polarization. It has focused on shared values rather than differences, presenting solutions that honor individual freedom, family, and community while respecting diverse perspectives. This commitment to unity underscores the belief that we are stronger when we work together toward common goals, even when we come from different viewpoints.

Each topic has been paired with practical actions—ways to make a difference at the local, state, and national levels. Whether supporting local businesses, engaging in civic discourse, advocating for fair policies, or simply sharing knowledge with others, the steps outlined in this book empower readers to translate their values into meaningful change. These actions demonstrate that everyone has the potential to contribute to a brighter future.

Ultimately, this book has envisioned a nation where opportunity is abundant, communities are safe and thriving, families are strong, and freedom is cherished. It's a vision of balance—where economic growth coexists with environmental stewardship, security is paired with compassion, and progress is rooted in tradition. This future isn't built by waiting for change but by each of us stepping forward, united by a shared commitment to the principles that guide us.

We have achieved a deeper understanding of the challenges and opportunities before us. We have embraced tools for personal growth and thoughtful engagement. We have fostered hope, resilience, and a belief that positive change is possible and within our reach. Most importantly, we have reaffirmed the values that define us, providing a pathway to strengthen ourselves and the communities and nations we hold dear.

This book is not the journey's end—it is a beginning. The conversations started here, the reflections prompted, and the actions inspired are all stepping stones toward a brighter tomorrow. Let us move forward with confidence, unity, and determination, carrying these principles into the world and the lives of those around us. Together, we can build a future where America's promise continues to shine, lighting the way for future generations.

www.ingramcontent.com/pod-product-compliance
Lightning Source LLC
Chambersburg PA
CBHW081547250726
48653CB00009B/3319